Lunar Abundance

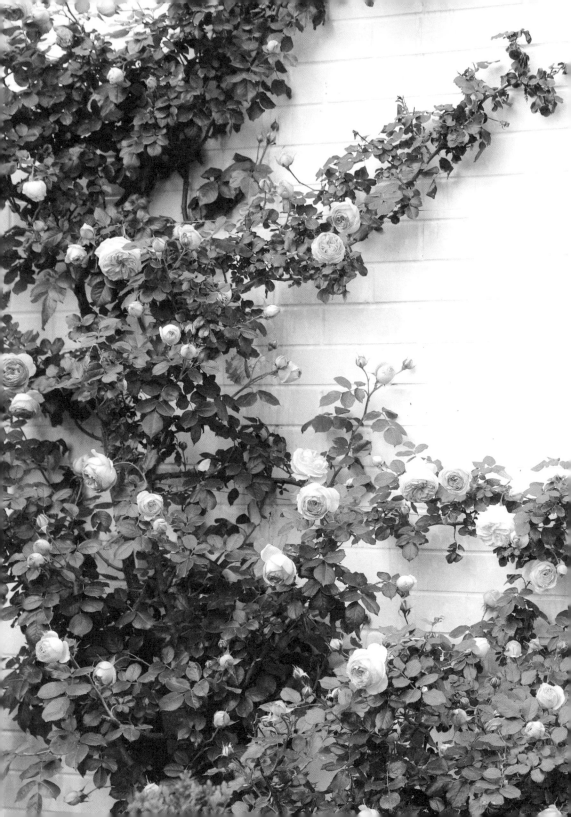

Lunar Abundance

CULTIVATING JOY, PEACE,
AND PURPOSE
USING THE PHASES OF THE MOON

Ezzie Spencer, PhD

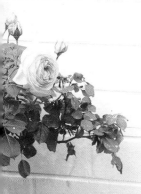

RUNNING PRESS
PHILADELPHIA

Running Press
Hachette Book Group
1290 Avenue of the Americas, New York, NY 10104
www.runningpress.com
@Running_Press

Printed in Canada

Originally published in 2017 by Xoum Publishing in Australia
First U.S. Edition: March 2018

Published by Running Press, an imprint of Perseus Books, LLC,
a subsidiary of Hachette Book Group, Inc.

The Hachette Speakers Bureau provides a wide range of authors for speaking events. To find out more, go to www.hachettespeakersbureau.com or call (866) 376-6591.

The publisher is not responsible for websites (or their content) that are not owned by the publisher.

Photography by Emma Kate Codrington and Andrew Moon.
Graphics by Sarah Gleeson.
Print book cover design by Ashley Todd.

Library of Congress Control Number: 2017953250

ISBNs: 978-0-7624-6357-2 (paperback), 978-0-7624-6356-5 (ebook)

FRI

10   9   8   7   6   5   4

To my fellow Moon gazers
around the Earth.

Contents

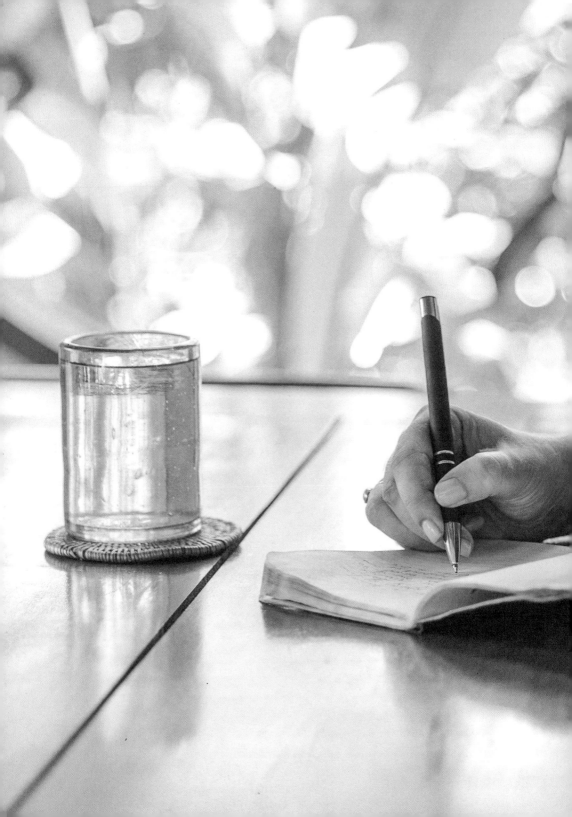

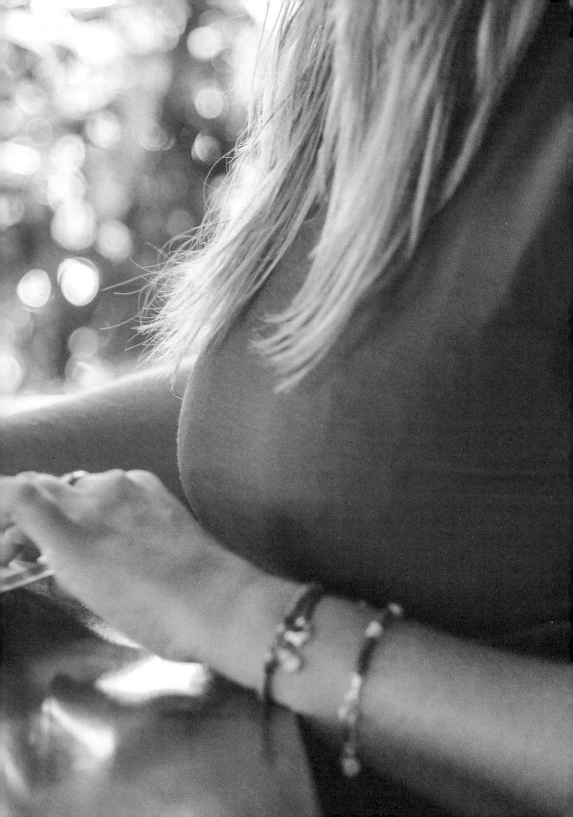

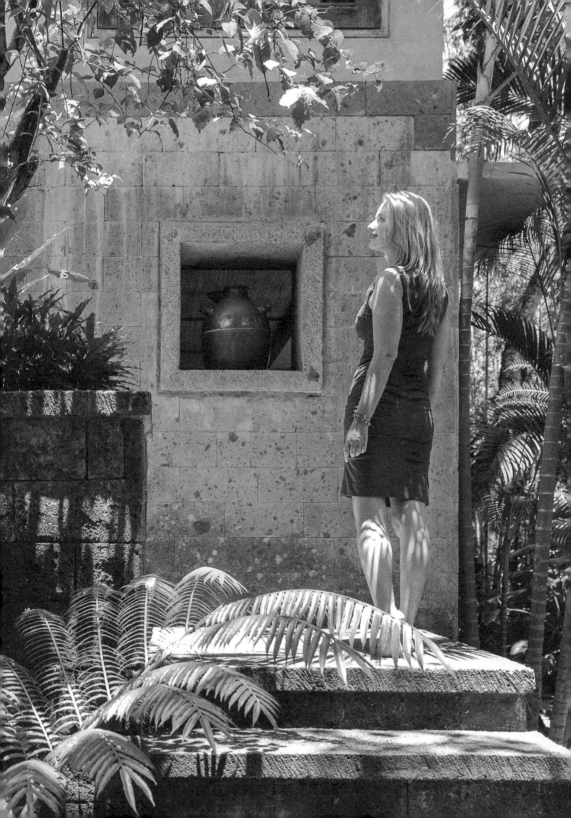

This Book Is For You If....

You are ready to get to know your own cycles, work in your natural flow, connect with something bigger and ride the accelerating waves of transformation and change on this planet.

It is for you if you are open to discovering a grounded, practical way to re-weave the gap between head and heart, mind and body; if you are ready to fully inhabit your own experience.

It is for you if you are ready to prosper and be well, to enjoy our precious time on this Earth, and give back to others from a place of abundance, rather than out of exhaustion, guilt, or fear.

If these words light you up, this book is ripe for your picking. It will help you summon your true potential, open your eyes to a better reality, and show you *how* to create a better life for you and for those in your orbit.

If you are ready to come home to yourself, and the rhythms of our exquisite world, here is your guidebook.

Lunar Abundance reveals this destination. It also sketches a map to navigate the journey.

There is a moon inside every human being.
Learn to be companions with it. [1]

—RUMI

To Begin

People often share with me their deeply felt connection with the Moon. Just looking at the Moon at night ignites our intuition and imagination, and evokes a *remembering* of sorts: an urge to pay attention.

We feel her ebb and flow; we feel her resonance with our own energy and physical cycles. We are intrigued by the mystique of her darkness and the climax of her light. We may also heed her call to transformation by tracking her rhythms: she offers a stability that speaks to our psyche in the ways she is always changing—ways that seem to be erratic, and yet are constant, cyclical, and predictable. She is elegant, romantic, and subtle. She represents both chaos and stability, a magnetic and mysterious riddle that draws us in with the possible richness in her depths. When we come closer, her links with fertility, bleeding, and creation reverberate in our bodies, hinting, too, at the nurturing and birth of our dreams.

Of course, interest in the Moon is not a phenomenon unique to the current social-media age. As one of Earth's luminaries, her lineage is ancient. This shining orb has captured the imagination of lovers and makers through the ages, and has inspired literature, poetry, song, and dance: all things creative and artisanal. The mythology of the Moon is found around the world, from the English namesake Luna in Rome to the Aztec Coyolxauhqui to Hina in Samoa. The Moon deities of many European, American, and Asian cultures tend to be female, but this is not exclusively the case, nor is it a consistent portrayal in all cultures. The female lunar archetypes are not all sweet and gentle, either, with goddesses that roar and devour, who are prone to matricide and infanticide and castration, as well as acts of creation and magic. Some are androgynous, some solemn forever-virgins, and others are depicted as routinely involved in incestuous copulation with bacchanalian fervor.

The inability of female goddesses, and even mythological women, to conform to gender stereotypes has long been confounding; Adam's first wife, Lillith, expressed a desire for equal partnership and the ability to enjoy an on-top sexual position and this led to her flight from the Garden of Eden into the clutches of demons, making way for a (somewhat) more pliant Eve—a patriarchy creation story not appearing in the Book of Genesis, but in the (satirical) Jewish text, the *Alphabet of Ben Sirah*, dated between 700–1000 CE. As those who come into closer relationship with the feminine know, it is not all flowing dresses in soft pink hues and flower crowns; the feminine can be *fierce*. Buddhist and Hindu traditions generally portray the goddesses as having both benign and terrifying aspects.[2] At times, the femme fatale can be the latter—Jane Caputi writes that this archetype "represents an outlawed form of female divinity, potency, genius, sexual agency, independence, vengeance and death power." The power of this face of the feminine is linked to ancient goddesses who regulate birth, life, death, change, and regeneration—the very cycle of existence.[3]

Is the Moon really about the "feminine"? It seems to have taken on that meaning in much of the West. "The feminine" is a slippery term to define. It is not the same thing as "female" or "woman"—but is it a concept, an archetype, a polarity, a kind of energy, a combination of these things, or something else entirely? In the West, the feminine tends to be associated with qualities or characteristics of what Simone de Beauvoir termed the Second Sex: feelings, emotion, flow, relationship, connection, nurturing, vulnerability, softness, receptivity, and intuition, to name a few. As essential aspects of the human condition, any person, regardless of gender, can express these characteristics. However, in the West, we allocate them primarily to the feminine, and while we can claim to cherish these, we have also devalued them in subtle or explicit

LUNAR ABUNDANCE

ways—a key one of these being the (lack of) financial value accorded to caring and healing-based work in capitalist societies that equate value with dollars.

If you accept that there is a resonance between the Moon and the feminine, it is not surprising that the Moon is experiencing an uptick in popularity in the West in parallel with the growing popularity of tradition-ally feminine qualities—collaboration over competition, soft power over force, Carol Gilligan's ethic of care.[4] Recent years have seen a surge in both leadership language and studies that indicate that we do, in fact, value intuition, emotional intelligence, vulnerability, community-building, inter-dependence, flexibility, and compassion.[5] Against the backdrop of both celebration and concern about the feminization of Western culture,[6] it is worth noting that some query the effectiveness of "feminine" values in a world that still reserves high rewards for reason, intellect, and cutthroat competition, and ask whether women are, in practice, disadvantaged by applying more "feminine" principles in leadership and work settings.[7] The debate illustrates that we have a way to travel yet, but I believe that harmonizing or balancing "masculine" and "feminine" qualities (and working toward gender equality) are worthy aspirations, and that decades of feminism have built a strong foundation upon which we may continue to build on both fronts.

When you reach the how-to parts of this book, you will find the term "Yin" refers specifically to the human "being" mode of operating (as opposed to the "Yang," or "doing," mode). Using these terms is my admittedly clumsy effort to create distance from gendered simplifications. There is a wealth of literature on Yin and Yang in the fields of Chinese medicine and relationships, which I do not

If you are interested, I encourage you to start to track the Moon, witness what happens with your own body, and make your mind up for yourself.

Free tracking resources available for download at www.lunarabundance.com

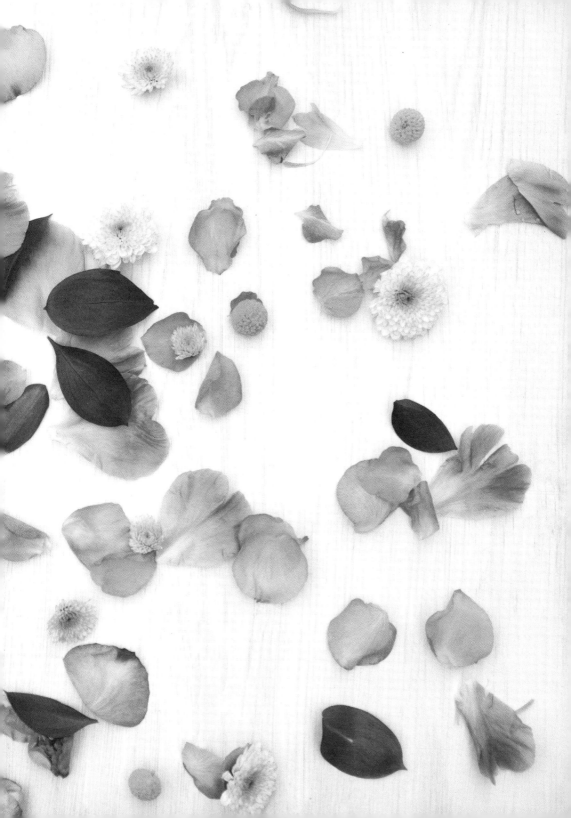

traverse in this book—the focus here is on the personal journey, and I refer to the terms Yin and Yang to reflect an inner alchemical process, as well as different modes of being and doing in the world. These terms are known well enough in English-speaking personal development circles to be meaningful, and are one way to avoid the sticky association between the terms feminine/woman and masculine/man, with the too-easy, essentialist claims to gender that accompany them (statements about how men and women "are" or "should be," often drawn uncritically from cultural stereotypes). Gender is complex,[8] but I believe we all need to *be* and *do* to be effective—and to enjoy life.

What I share in these pages is my personal practice: how to work with the Moon, her monthly cycles, and the eight phases within each. This book is based on the knowledge that I have gained by sharing this practice with thousands of women online, in-depth with women in several countries, and with occasionally interested men. I believe that regulating our lives through observation of the Moon—the practice I call "Lunar Abundance"—contains universal wisdom about the Yin mode of being (and about finding harmony between the Yin and Yang modes of operating) and can offer guidance to those who do not share my identity or experience. I do, though, identify as a cis-gendered woman who experiences the intersection of race, class, and so forth in ways that are to my benefit, and as I was the guinea pig for this practice, I tend to teach and write from my own perspective.[9]

We are all free to look up at night and gaze at the Moon—humans have been working with the Moon for eons. Many of us in the modern world worry about whether we are "doing it right," and yet there is no one way to do it. I work with the Moon as a natural timekeeper, in the pursuit of peace and effectiveness.

While not the exclusive domain of women, there does seem to be an affinity between the Moon and women's bodies—most obviously, our menstrual cycle. Notches in bone calendars from 35,000 BCE marked Moon and menstrual phases.[10] Though Aristotle wrote off the connection between the Moon and menstrual cycles as coincidence thousands of years ago,[11] many a woman who starts to work with the Moon has written to me in order to share how the practice has resulted in welcome physical changes for her body. Those who have experienced a long pause may start to bleed again; those with irregular cycles may start to experience greater regularity; for some, discomfort while bleeding has even given way to pleasure—something that I personally know is physically possible, if not the stereotype. If you bleed, and you find that following the Moon has a positive impact on your bleeding and associated symptoms, know that you are not alone.

I am not a medical doctor—if you have concerns about your body, please seek professional care. However, I do know that gaining knowledge of your menstrual cycle seems to enhance women's well-being. On this, I encourage you to explore the work of Dr. Christiane Northrup, Miranda Gray, and several others listed in the Resources section at the back of this book. I also cannot ignore that women from all over the world write to tell me over and over that tuning into the Moon has been impactful, meaningful, and helpful for them in connecting to their menstrual cycle. Given histories of shame, fear, and disparagement around the menstruation process—as with so much to do with the female body—I believe that when women speak their own truth about their bodies, we must listen with openness, and respond with curiosity by asking further questions. Note that the benefits of following the Moon cycle can be felt regardless of whether you are menstruating or not.

The Moon is quintessentially coupled with our emotional and feeling terrain. I use the term "feelings" to mean physical sensations, and "emotions" to mean surges of fear, anger, love, desire—the *meaning* that we accord to what we *feel*. In this lunar practice, I am most interested in feelings, as these are the pathway to embodiment, but feelings and emotions are indeed linked, and the Moon relates to both. Most who pay attention can particularly feel their own heightened sensitivity to feelings and emotions under the Full Moon phase. Workers in the justice, health, or childhood education sectors are usually the first to agree, vigorously, that this Moon phase is a time of intensity; a stirring-up. Several studies document that humans sleep at least a little less under the Full Moon,[12] and a smattering of studies indicate that crime[13] and hospitals[14] see heightened activity at this Moon phase. Of course, plenty of researchers have set out to debunk the "Full Moon myth," but in turn, some countervailing studies have been criticized on the basis of specific definitions of what counts as the Full Moon phase.[15]

Our understanding of the relevance of the Moon in our lives on Earth is embedded in the English language. We need only return to the roots of the English word "lunacy" to see that we have long known about some kind of relationship between the Moon and our lives down below on Earth. Lunacy did not always have a negative connotation; in *Mysteries of the Dark Moon*, Demetra George explains that the ancient Greek triple Moon goddess Hekate bestowed lunacy as a temporary quality upon chosen recipients to facilitate vision, prophetic insight, and magical powers.[16] We also know that there is something romantic about the Moon: to be "moony" is to gaze with soft eyes in love.

Why does the Moon have the effect that it does? Do we actually know? In *Moonstruck: How Lunar Cycles Affect Life*, Ernest Naylor explains how scientists tend to avoid research into lunar cycles for the reason that its links with "irrationality" would sound the death knell on a respectable scientific career. There are theories, though. For example, as the Moon affects the ocean tides, and because we have a significant amount of water in our own bodies, the gravitational pull of the Moon may also affect the human body and psyche. This is often refuted by the scientific community, but those who have been close to the epicenter of a total solar eclipse—occurring when the orbits of the Earth, Moon, and Sun align in a certain way—have spoken to me of the exhilarating and cathartic nature of this experience, which is also documented to affect the environment through changes in wind direction, as well as in temperature.[17] Solar eclipses can be so profound for those who experience them that there is a name for those who follow eclipses from remote Arctic seas to the Australian desert, from bustling metropolises to sites of political instability: umbraphiles.

Or the relationship may not be cause-and-effect after all. Dr. Carl Jung suggested that we experience celestial entities through synchronicity: meaningful coincidence, acausal connection, or—as the ancient Hermetic principle of correspondence would have it—*as above, so below*.[18] With this reading, the relationship becomes one of correlation, or representation. To see the Moon as reflective is a neat fit: as the Moon reflects the light of the Sun in the sky, it also reflects this back to us on Earth. We experience an illumination of what is represented by the Moon—our own emotional terrain—which can be disorienting if we are not equipped with the tools to respond.

You do not need to closely follow the Moon to experience synchronicity, but greater attention does seem to enhance the effects. Thus, there may be another reason that following the Moon phases has the effect that it does: *us*. Our very gaze may imbue the Moon cycle with meaning for ourselves. At the edge of quantum physics, scientists have shown that reality does not exist until it is measured: the object of our attention is influenced by the very fact that we are paying attention to it.[19] This may be one of the reasons why the Lunar Abundance practice is effective. In fact, I believe that most things that help you pay attention to your internal world will help you cultivate self-knowledge, which in turn will help you skillfully navigate the external world. This is important, as the inner work is not an end in and of itself.

As there have been many opinions but not comprehensive research, to date, on why the Moon has the effect that it does, I feel most comfortable describing my engagement with the Moon less through blind faith, and more through the act of natural timekeeping and conscious awareness.

Why is this valuable? The more you know yourself, the less you are influenced by external forces; the more you are able to hear your own deep wisdom and embrace your true nature—who you are, where you belong, and which way is the right direction—in order to take discerning action.

The Moon cycle is what continually guides me home and grounds me; she was my initial inspiration, remains my muse, and provides, via her short, trackable, and observable cycle, a gentle and predictable rhythm and guide to situate myself here on Earth, as well as a mirror back to us to help us know ourselves. The Moon has helped me to cultivate a more intimate integration of mind and body, and to devise a rule-of-thumb guide for living and working in my own flow. With this, I create a better life for myself and for those with whom I share this practice.

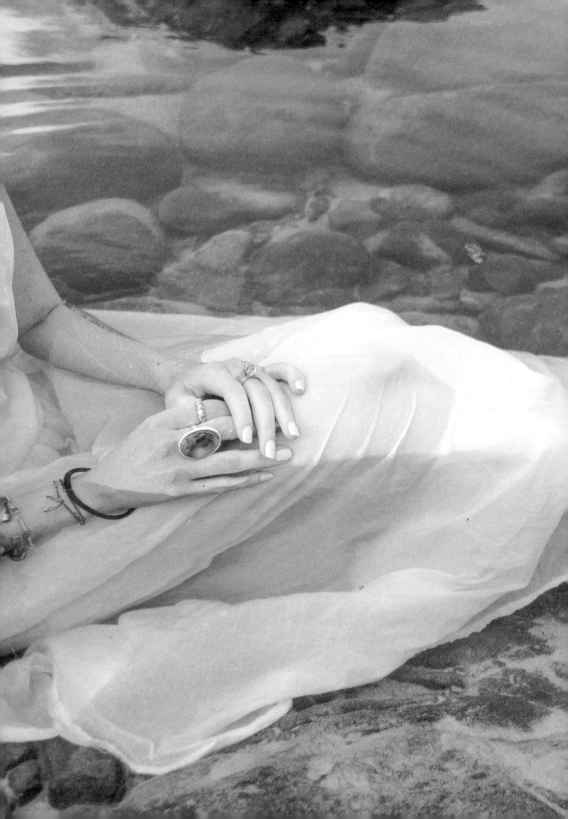

The more you *know yourself,*

the less you are influenced by

external forces;

the more you are able to hear

your own *deep wisdom* and

embrace your *true nature* —

who you *are,* where you *belong,*

and which way is the *right direction* —

in order to take discerning action.

I definitely do not suggest that the Moon makes us do anything—how disempowering would that be? Throughout this book, I show you how to work with the Moon cycle in my way, and to explore what the Moon has guided me to learn: our own rhythms and cycles, the contours of our creative power, the natural ebb and flow of work and life, the necessity of self-care and connection with all that is physical and real—as well as the interplay between the night and day, the shadow and the light, the ups and downs inherent in life. We need the Moon to function here on Earth, even if we do not always pay her as much attention as we do the Sun.

In uncertain and changing times, it can be helpful to find our anchor in both self-knowledge and a supportive community. By self-knowledge, I am not referring to fanciful thinking, to compulsive worry, or to "realizations" fueled by commodified sacred arts skillfully marketed to our subconscious vulnerabilities. I am talking about those times when we *know* something to be true: those times when our heart and gut speak to us—when we physically feel it. That we should not get in that car. That there is something amiss in our body. That our friend suddenly needs help. That he seems so nice, and our friends and family think we are being too picky, but we should end our relationship with that man. Or that we need to make that big change—even though it seems inconvenient at best, and terrifying at worst.

How can you tell the difference? The magic answer: it takes time, practice, and a deep knowing of yourself and your place in the world. The practices in this book are designed to show you how to cultivate the ability to hear, honor, respect, trust, and then act upon your own knowing.

This book reveals this *destination*.

It also sketches a *map*

to *navigate* the journey.

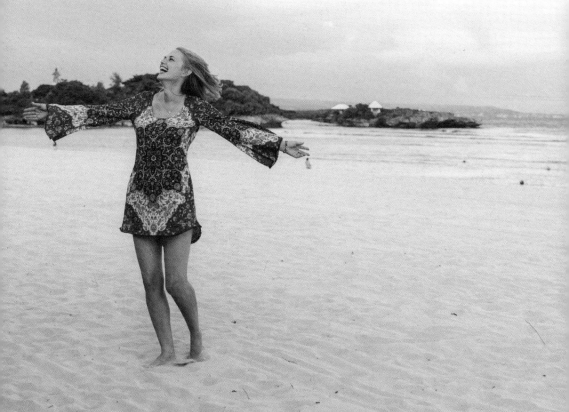

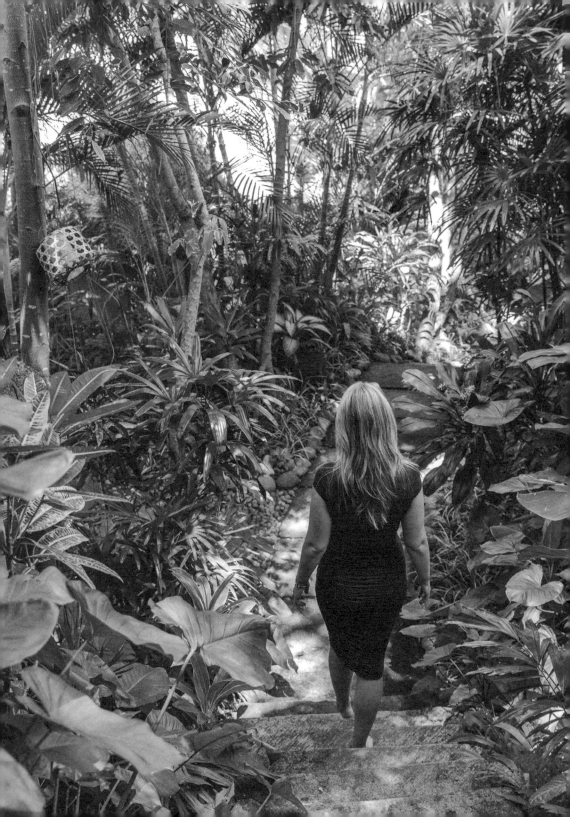

How This All Came About

Lunar Abundance is a practice that will help you cultivate peace, self-knowledge, effectiveness, stability, trust, and flow by following the Moon cycle, in a very safe, contained and gently transformative process.

Are these qualities actually inherent to the Moon? Symbolic correlations exist, but as this is my personal interpretation of how to work with the Moon cycle, rather than a "this is the way to work with the Moon" manifesto, you may like to know more about me in order to understand a little more about how and why I developed this practice.

I've always been quietly fascinated by the Moon. I had that sense of something bigger than myself as a child: a connection to other worlds, a fascination with the esoteric and ancient times, with myth and magic. This sense of mystery faded into the background once I decided to go to law school, which I saw as a ticket to a bright future. Once at law school, I found that the clarity of its systems and its intellectual rigor gave me access to bold claims about objective reality. My brain was pushed, pulled, and tested beyond its limits when surrounded day in and day out by kind, thoughtful, and deep thinkers at a school where the baseline was excellence. I was a tiny goldfish among the koi, summoning the A-type elements of my personality to the forefront to succeed.

I was trained to see the law as a powerful vehicle through which to effect social justice, and upon graduation was thrilled to land work in a government agency that reviewed federal laws to ensure that they were modern, effective, just, and in line with Australia's human rights obligations. My law work was meaningful and enabled me to give back to those less privileged than myself; I worked with inspiring colleagues and leaders.

While I did not know what was absent, I sensed that I was missing something. An accident when I was 22 years old—a simple fall down stairs resulted in a shattered left knee and major reconstructive surgeries—sent me down the path of somatic therapies throughout my twenties and beyond, providing me with the first hints that I was out of touch with my body, both before and after the accident. The busy worlds of study and work had provided a welcome sanctuary from feeling much at all. I slowly went further and found that I was disconnected from my own cycles, as well as the needs and potential of my female body. This is not unusual: Tracy Gaudet and Paula Spencer suggest that many women are "unconsciously female," with external influences such as a diet culture and cultural objectification of women preventing an early establishment of intimacy with our own physical selves.[20]

Inhabiting the very heady and intellectual world of the law by day, I would explore the sense of something missing at night by journaling. I started to notice where the Moon was at night, drawing a little picture of the phase in my journal entries. Over some Moon cycles, I noticed patterns emerging: I observed correlations between how I was feeling and what phase the Moon was in. This was utterly fascinating, and from this starting place I began to work more consciously with the Moon and with what was being revealed to me. I started to open up, at first slowly and then rapidly over time, as I began to comprehend that there was more to reality—and life—than what I had perceived up to this point.

For someone who had lived from the neck up in many ways, I started to find that my female body could be an ongoing site of pleasure, of wisdom, and of personal power, rather than something that I had to take care of at best, or something that let me down at worst. As my lunar practice evolved, my own cycles became a source of pleasure and personal power. My creativity and productivity sky-rocketed when I gave myself the space to draw back, restore, and reflect when my body asked, rather than mindlessly pushing forward. Amid the inevitable oscillations of life, my reality started to evolve in other ways, too: my friendship circles started to expand dramatically at a time of life when they were meant to be shrinking; my relationships with others became deeper and more fulfilling; my physical energy levels rose; my hope in, love of, and trust in life grew; I became less afraid to express my thoughts and desires; my self-esteem deepened. I became more present—and felt more alive.

Tuning into the needs of my body and feelings—the physical sensations in my body—was key to this, and in Lunar Abundance, the Moon represents the feelings. However, in bringing feelings to the forefront, I have not

Inhabiting the very heady and intellectual world of the law by day, I would explore the sense of something missing at night by journaling.

Free lunar journaling resources available for download at www.lunarabundance.com

abandoned the thinking mind. I believe that enhanced personal potency and well-being come from the marriage of feelings and rational thought, mind and body, Yin and Yang, intellect and intuition, and subjectivity and objectivity. My respect for rigorous thought remains, and informs my ongoing desire to integrate head and heart.

Eventually, I left a secure and traditional career, which I had liked, for one that felt more creative and richly fulfilling, as well as more suited to my growing strengths. But this was a slow burn. As I tracked the Moon at night throughout my twenties, I continued to evolve my original career by day. With the encouragement of a wonderful mentor, I sidestepped into legal academia to teach when I was 28 and completed a PhD in women's well-being when seeking justice after sexual violence, an issue that had inflamed me while working in law reform. And, no longer working defined hours, I started to find my own flow: taking my lunar practice to the next level as I went deeper into understanding my own cycles, and aligning these with the Yin and Yang phases of the Moon (an aspect of the lunar practice that I explain over the coming chapters). My thesis poured out as I found that I was far more effective when following my own rhythms, harnessing my growing knowledge about when to push forward and when to relax and restore.

Enhanced productivity, together with a flexible researcher schedule, also opened space on my calendar to share my more intuitive work with others, creating a side income through client sessions. Continuing on with public policy and research work in the women's safety sector after finishing my doctorate, I eventually moved into full-time creative entrepreneurship when it became apparent to me that my side interests were changing me irrevocably, and the call to immerse myself in these was too strong to ignore. Facilitating transformation directly in women's lives (and having fun while doing it!) is where I feel fully in my element.

I have not traced a linear path to where I am now; it took many Moon cycles for the seeds planted in those early client sessions to bear fruit. I nurtured these without assurance of how they might grow, learning how to better cultivate patience and allow uncomfortable uncertainty to become part of my life as I followed the crumbs to where I am now. As you will discover in many of the Yin Moon phases, being *with* the inherent uncertainty of life—rather than rushing to fill the pauses by "keeping busy"—is a core part of the lunar practice, and is essential in unlocking the magic of a life that honors both Yin and Yang.

The Lunar Abundance practice emerged as I learned from teachers and guides whom I mention throughout this book, as well as experimentation and sharing my practices with thousands of others, with a curiosity as to how it plays. From a meta-perspective, the Lunar Abundance practice is informed by my understanding of lunar cycles, elements of Taoism, Jungian individuation (in the sense of the quest for wholeness), desire for self-actualization, embodiment, and a sense of universal responsibility. While I meditate daily and feel connected to a bigger—nameless—something, I do not belong to a specific spiritual lineage or religious tradition, although my family of origin is (nonpracticing) Protestant, and no doubt this, together with my Australian upbringing, has shaped much of how I see the world in ways that I have not fully identified or deconstructed. I aim, at least, to be both effective and ethical, and see the means existing in relation to the ends—I believe that both are important. I believe that you can be deeply intuitive and connected to your internal, subjective world, and still grounded in objective reality. Maybe I am most of all a pragmatist: a modern woman in the world seeking love and growth, connection and camaraderie, joy and abundance. I want to give back where I can and I also want to enjoy my time here on Earth. This is what drives me.

If you have access to resources that allow you to be an agent of change in your life's narrative, then this book is an exhortation to make the most of it. It includes practical steps to help you enjoy your bounty, release the struggle, and share the love. I hope, too, that there are universal truths in this book that involve tapping into your own intuition and wisdom, honoring your body, and connecting with others, all of which are foundational to creating a better life, regardless of your starting point.

The Moon wisdom in this book is offered to you in this spirit.

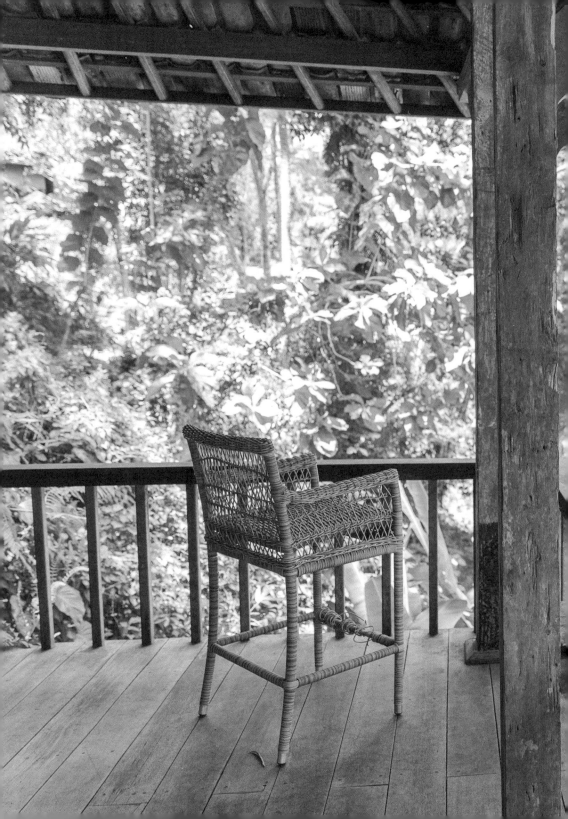

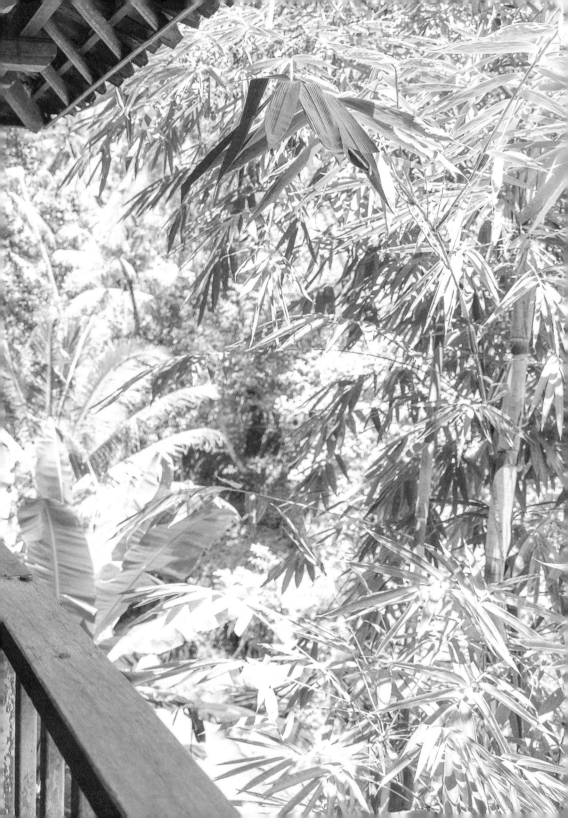

The psyches and souls of women also have
their own cycles and seasons of doing and solitude,
running and staying, being involved and being removed,
questing and resting, creating and incubating,
being of the world and returning to the soul-place.[21]

—DR. CLARISSA PINKOLA ESTÉS

Cycles and Phases
of the Moon

Cycles can be found throughout all of life: the Moon around the Earth, yes, but also the Earth's cycle around the Sun (and the cycles of all celestial bodies); the cycle of the day; the cycle of the seasons; cycles of plants; cycles of birds' and animals' migration and hunting.

Within our bodies we have the circadian rhythm, and cycles of our immune, endocrine, and nervous systems. In our mundane world, we have the cycles of the market and economic development. In the spiritual dimension, in cultures that believe in reincarnation, death is followed by life and, again, death. Despite the omnipresence of cycles, Western culture celebrates a linear conception of time and life, in a way that Rebecca Orleane suggests is a bid to control our natural environment, and inhibits our awareness of these flowing patterns that are inherent to our life here on Earth.[22]

This book is a gateway through which to remember the ubiquity of cycles, and it shows you how to embed *one* cycle into your life; to work with the Moon cycle in a way that is meaningful for you. The Moon cycle takes about a month, and within that cycle, the Moon moves through eight phases of a few days apiece. These eight Moon phases are in fact co-created by the orbits of the Moon, Earth, and Sun. The Moon takes about a month to orbit the Earth, and the sunlight that the Moon reflects to Earth in each of the eight phases within that month is a result of the Moon's position in relation to the Sun. Each of the following chapters of this book is based on one of the eight Moon phases, starting at the New Moon. Each of the phases (or chapters) builds on the last, waxing with a crescendo to the Full Moon and waning back to the New Moon. The cycle then repeats; the invitation is to revisit these chapters and phases in each Moon cycle, moving ever deeper into the practice.

You will get the most out of this book if you have an existing curiosity about the Moon and already want to make changes in your life, but are not sure exactly what this would look like in practice. Opining on how you *should* lead your life or why you *should* look at the Moon does not turn me on. If you are not interested in the Moon cycle, that is perfectly fine—my project is not to convince you of its relevance. Equally, if you do not want to change your life, I am not here to proselytize or suggest that you should be doing things better. This book is a very practical guide on how to create a better life, intended to meet you at a point when you are seeking this, and especially when you are curious about the Moon cycle and phases. It can be a complement for a spiritual tradition if you have one, but you do not need a spiritual connection to include this practice in your everyday life. It is a way to help you create a better version of your own life, with results that you can see.

When does the next Moon cycle start?

Free lunar planner resources available for download at www.lunarabundance.com

To underscore: this lunar practice can be effective without suggesting that the Moon *makes* us do anything. We work with the Moon as a natural timekeeper, a method to track a deep dive into ourselves, and a natural calendar for us to engage more with our world and spirituality, if this is relevant for us. And if you are not sure whether it is for you—give it a go and decide for yourself.

Practices are experienced and felt, they garner results through process, and they become a way of life. Practices involve devotion and commitment, as well as consistency and repetition, and those who persevere will see cumulative effects over time.

The Lunar Abundance practice contained in this book focuses first on connection to self, others, and the broader world, and second, on creating a more abundant life.

There is a coming home and reconnection in the first level of practice: self-knowledge and embodiment, a connection to community, Earth, and beyond.

This practice helps us to see ourselves, to be compassionate with what we find, and to remember who we really are. In line with the principle of correspondence, the Moon acts as a trigger for us to look within. When we glance up at night to see her, she mirrors us back to ourselves. She anchors us in our world by reminding us always to move our gaze within. In this way, she is a consistent and reliable guide to remind us to tune into ourselves, to feel our bodies, to witness and then flow with our own natural rhythms. Working with the Moon cycle in the way that I set out in this book is one way to cultivate self-knowledge—connection with the self.

Beyond connection with ourselves, we may also seek camaraderie with one another—dissolving our wounds with women and connecting with one another in a way that is genuinely supportive and lifts each of us higher. It is a way to overcome loneliness, to build healthy relationships, to collaborate and create something powerful and inviting. We can develop this through joining together in New Moon and Full Moon practices, as well as by cultivating the qualities of relating and giving back, which are essential aspects of this lunar practice.

The connection that we seek moves beyond the human form. In casting her gaze back down to Earth, the Moon's light nudges many of us to remember our connection to our natural environment. We sense the discomfort of our Earth in watching the storms that come with increasing frequency and ferocity, snow at odd times of the year, and winters that seem too warm. We feel disconnected from something important: from the sites where our food is grown, from the treatment of animals, from the bosom of the Great Mother herself. Attention alone will not solve the issues of our planet, but it will help to reconnect us with the ground that provides us with support, nourishment, and life, and will set the stage for more work in this area.

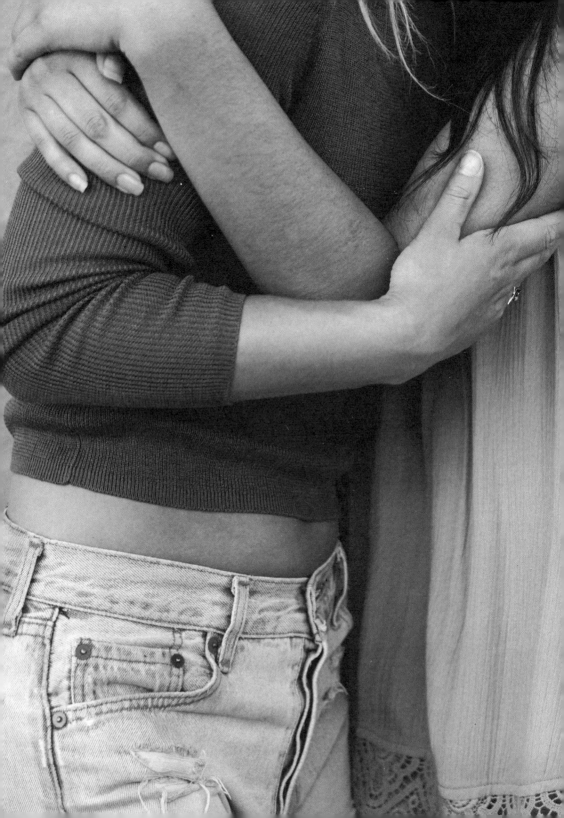

The *practice* contained
in this book focuses, first,
on connection to *self, others,*
and the *broader world,*
and, second, on creating
a *more abundant life.*

Some of us also crave a connection with something bigger again. As the Moon catches our eye of an evening, we catch a tiny glimpse of the universe expanding beyond, and we are reminded of what exists beyond our own small world. There is a void that many ache to fill: another disconnection to which we feel that we must attend, even if we cannot put words around what is missing. The rise in the popularity of meditation in the West in recent years—part of this lunar practice—also speaks to this need for greater connection: both to the soul and something far greater, however defined.

Throughout this book, you will get to know some of my clients who make their way through the practice at different levels. These are real people with real experiences with the lunar practice. All stories are shared with permission, with some names and features changed to protect their privacy.

The Moon offers us a mirror for self-awareness, as well as a path on which to practice self-care and enhance our well-being. The Moon offers even more than this: she offers us a way to cultivate greater abundance. When I refer to "abundance," I'm not just using this as a synonym for money—and certainly do not mean greed or excess. I mean it as a way of being, of living in the overflow (with certain thoughts, and actions, flowing from this in turn)—a way to invite more goodness into your life. Once you develop a deep understanding of abundance, and start to act in accordance with this understanding, my experience has been that more of *everything* will flow. But it's not about striving: abundance involves gentle steeping in self-love and trusting in the right process.

Examples of abundance include more rest, more energy to do what needs to get done, and a greater sense of well-being. Abundance is about freeing yourself from anxiety about what you don't have, living in a relaxed way where you know that you will have enough. Abundance is about peace as much as it is about prosperity. And, one way to cultivate abundance is to practice.

Working in a very specific way with the Moon cycle, which I explain in these pages, has helped me to practice this. It has also helped me to practice *being*; to be kind with myself and allow success by rest and pacing, rather than by relentless striving. My own shadow pattern is to push myself to burnout—or the brink of it.

Time and time again I have been to this place, with my body reacting with illness and usually, also, a flare-up of my chronic injury to signal the need to slow down. Many successful women share this shadow, which is caused partly by a genuine love of our craft, and partly by a perfectionism fueled by "imposter syndrome" and our inner critic, a sense of not being good enough, and a fear that if we do not push ourselves to the nth degree we will *fail*, resulting in the symbolic death of our identity, if not the literal form.

There are other very good reasons, of course, for why women work hard. We are also driven by exigencies of modern life: the boundaries of work and life are increasingly permeable, while life and children and other family responsibilities require us to keep multiple plates spinning, and financial instability and debt can require ever more hours. Let's not forget that unconscious bias is an actual thing, women face the double bind in workplaces, and as Annabel Crabb notes, most institutional careers are still based on the assumption that there is a wife at home, with women who cannot afford to hire someone for that role still finding it harder than men to find a romantic partner to play it for them.[23]

In other words, working hard is not always a choice.

I bring up these structural issues because they are real, and cannot be remedied through a changed mind-set and individual choice alone. Structural inequality, or the social and political forces that shape our world, extend well beyond gender, of course—gender always intersects with elements such as race, class, and physical ability—sometimes to the benefit and sometimes to the detriment of those involved, although we know that certain combinations always tend to fall to the lower end of hierarchies of privilege. If you dream of becoming a millionaire and choose to pursue this via the Lunar Abundance practice, it does not mean that structural inequalities will cease to be obstacles; you do not need to internalize this as a personal failing, or see it as a failing of the practice. The lunar practice in this book is designed to help you reframe your approach to life, to help you explore those pockets where you *do* have agency, and to exercise it. Beyond that, I believe that it is about playing a better hand with the cards you were dealt *and* aiming to change the game: a both/and strategy rather than an either/or.

This practice is designed to help women in the Yang way of life who want to slow down to experience more Yin. At times I explain how to effectively work with Yang Moon phases to overcome resistance, procrastination, fear, and doubt; however, the Lunar Abundance practice is specifically directed toward helping those who find it difficult to turn off—rather than those who need help switching on—and who experience deleterious effects on well-being as a result.

I do not suggest slowing down simply because it is nice to relax, by the way: I suggest that slowing down is a necessary component of a life where our brain has the time that it needs to process important information, and where we reduce mental and emotional stress, and avoid physical burnout, while still getting the important things done.[24] I had to bring about changes to make my ongoing productivity tenable, and to shape a life conducive to physical and emotional well-being. Well-being is inherently subjective. For me, it means being healthy, energized, and (generally) calm rather than constantly stressed. Consider your own definition, and work toward cultivating it with this practice.

EIGHT CHAPTERS

What you will find in this book is a manual, a how-to, and a way for you to start to work effectively with the Moon cycle yourself, whether you engage with it as a Lunar Abundance practice or not.

There are eight practical chapters in this book, outlined below. Each aligns with one of the eight Moon phases. In each chapter—so, in each Moon phase—you can engage with each of the levels set out above. Throughout each chapter, you will find questions for inquiry to help you engage with each of these levels. At the end of the Moon cycle, you return to the New Moon, which is an opportunity to revisit the exercises and go deeper again.

With her rolling cycle, the Moon speaks to me of the essence of abundance. She won't "run out." You will not "miss it." You can't miss it: she is there for you when you are ready. There will be another New Moon, another cycle, and another opportunity for you to engage with the wisdom of the Moon cycle.

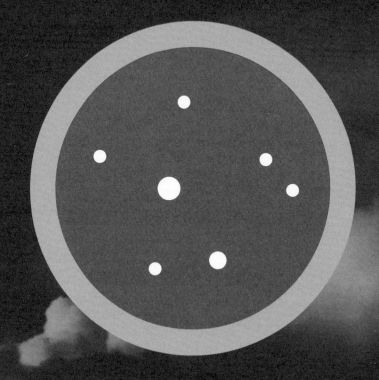

NEW MOON

The New Moon occurs when the Moon is dark in the sky—the very beginning of
the cycle. In the New Moon chapter, you will learn how to go within to reconnect
with yourself. We will explore the power of *intention*.

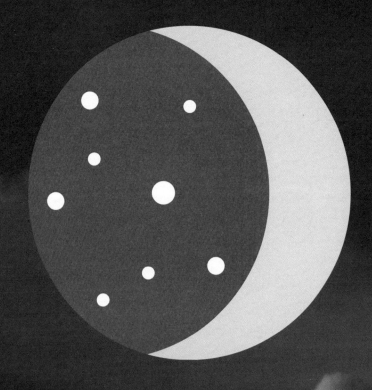

CRESCENT MOON

There is now some light in the sky. In the Crescent Moon chapter, you will be introduced to the essential nature of the Yin phases.

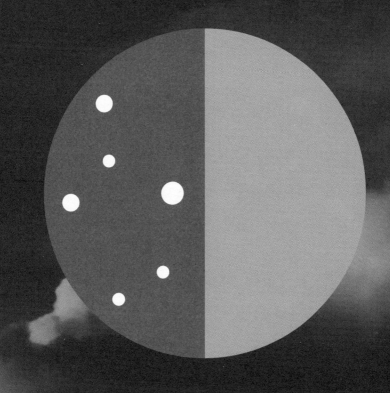

FIRST QUARTER MOON

In the First Quarter Moon chapter, we will continue the theme of reconnection with our self, seeing how self-knowledge can inform discernment. As the second Yang phase, we will understand more about what Yang phases really are, and also see what discernment looks like in daily action.

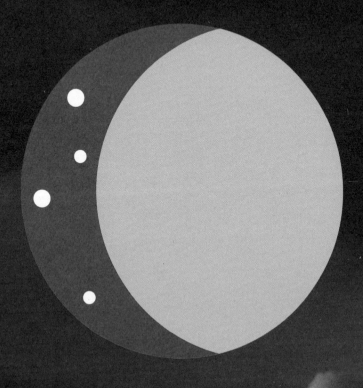

GIBBOUS MOON

The Moon is now waxing to Full—but it is not there yet. In the Gibbous Moon chapter, we will answer some sticky questions about the Yin phases: What does "being" look like in practice? We will also explore the principle of trust.

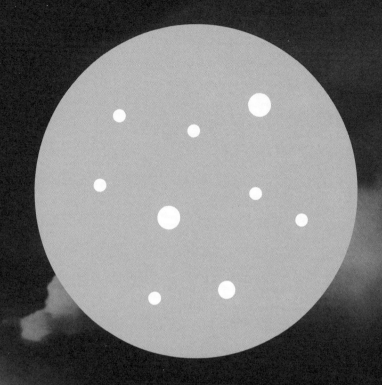

FULL MOON

The time of illumination and emotional climax. In the Full Moon chapter, we will explore reconnection with our own emotions and inner world. We will also discuss how to charge ahead with the Yang phase, or to change direction if we are off course. We will also explore the principle of letting go.

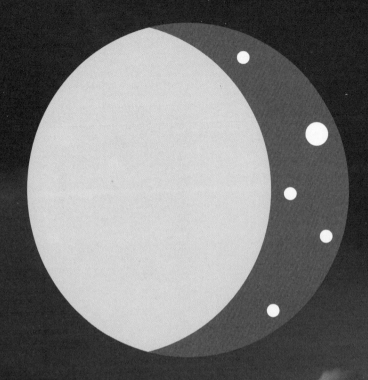

DISSEMINATING MOON

In this chapter, we will start to reconnect with our self—specifically, our own self-worth. We also explore what the Yin phase may have to offer us outside of work. We will explore receiving and gratitude—what these principles are, and aren't.

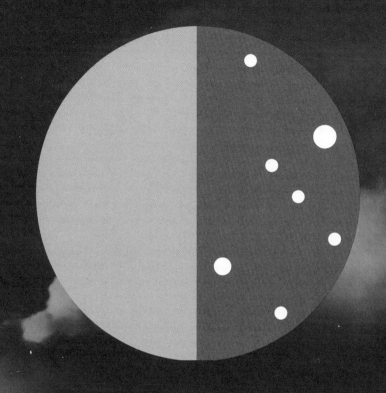

THIRD QUARTER MOON

In this chapter, we will explore reconnection with the Earth. It is also the final push, so we explore how Yang phases can help us overcome fear. We explore the principle of giving back.

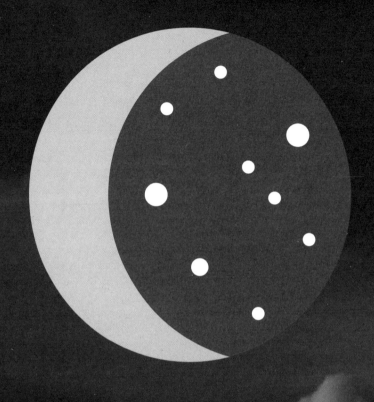

BALSAMIC MOON

The Moon is fading to dark. In this phase, we explore a connection to something much bigger. We also explore how Yin goes beyond baths and yoga to deep reflection and restoration.

If you wish to come back home to yourself, to create the conditions of well-being, and to become an agent of change in your own life's narrative, then engage with the practice laid out in these chapters. Think, for sure, but also carry out the exercises and feel, for it is the embodiment of the Lunar Abundance principles that will help you to find richness in the flow of the Moon.

Without further ado . . .

let's begin.

Each New Moon

Set a thematic, positive, feeling-based
intention for that lunar cycle.

Make it just about you.

Create a Life of Abundance

Create a life of abundance by *doing* certain things at Yang lunar

phases; and *being* a certain way at Yin lunar phases.

NEW MOON {YANG}
I set my intention. I feel my intention in my body.

CRESCENT MOON {YIN}
I relax into my intention. I breathe.

FIRST QUARTER MOON {YANG}
I take discerning action to support my intention.

GIBBOUS MOON {YIN}
I trust that the perfect intention is coming into form at the perfect time.

FULL MOON {YANG}
I move ahead with my intention now, OR I accept that my intention was not for the best at this time. I release it, and course-correct now.

DISSEMINATING MOON {YIN}
I feel grateful that my intention is coming into form in the perfect way. I receive with gratitude.

THIRD QUARTER MOON {YANG}
Now that I am receiving my intention, I give back from a place of abundance.

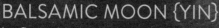

BALSAMIC MOON {YIN}
I reflect with thanks. I rest. I restore.

Who looks outside dreams, who looks inside awakes.[25]

—DR. CARL JUNG

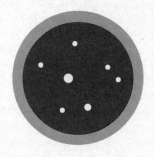

New Moon

As we move through the motions of the day, we may catch sight of the Moon in the afternoon or evening.

There she is, on our drive home after work or from our porch or back garden; her majestic glow evokes a feeling that can be ephemeral and difficult to pin down, but nevertheless feels important. She evokes that feeling of security via her constancy, pinned to the sky.

At the exact moment of the New Moon, though, there is little light to catch sight of. In fact, the first of the eight Moon phases is when the Moon is barely discernible in the sky. You can see her outline if you focus your eyes in the right direction during the day as the New Moon rises and sets with the Sun—it is in line with the Sun, after all—and slowly, a sliver of light starts to emerge. The Moon cycle starts in proverbial darkness as the Moon moves between the Earth and the Sun, blocking the Sun's rays from our view.

This darkness is the reference point from which we begin our journey through the Moon phases. Why? When you are in darkness, stripped of visual cues, you are steered toward the well of wisdom that lies within. Steering within in this way is how we access the rich symbolic soil of this first lunar phase.

Our souls are longing for this reconnection with the natural rhythms of our world. When we are away from all the physical comforts of the city, allowing us to reconnect with the Earth, we become able to feel how good that reconnection can be.

We often avoid the dark because it is uncomfortable and unknown. Yet it is in the darkness that we can start to uncover our hidden riches.

As Dr. Azita Nahai says, *"The only way is through."* And the way *through* is to *feel*.

RECONNECTING TO FEELINGS

At the New Moon, in the metaphorical darkness, our visual senses—together with the senses of hearing, touch, taste, and smell—help us to navigate a three-dimensional world. And yet we also have the ability to feel without touch, to engage with what author and healer Kevin Farrow calls *the feeling sense*.[26] While our imaginings can be a useful starting point, bodily feelings or sensations are the gateway to a world that is richer than the imagination.

When I refer to feelings here, I mean physical sensations—which, as Kevin Farrow teaches, emanate from an open heart. When I speak of feelings, I do not encourage prejudice or unconscious bias at the expense of thought. Make no mistake: your ability to think is one of your greatest assets, and as you will find, this practice encourages you to think for yourself: to cultivate truth and wisdom.

But when we are interested in coming home to ourselves, to explore the borders of reality that are starting to shift and change—when our mind has guided us this far, we realize that thinking is not the full picture. Thinking often gives us the impression that we are going somewhere, or that we are inhabiting a place that we are not. It might give us the impression that we are important, wonderful, awful, spiritual, fat, skinny, right, stupid, smart, advanced, the best, the worst, or perhaps all of the above in the space of an hour.

Our thinking might also give us the impression that this is the sum total of reality, that this is what life is. It is not. There is more. To go deeper, start to experience, rather than merely intellectualizing. And the easiest way to start to experience life is to feel. There is nothing imagined about feeling: it is palpable and real. You literally feel what is going on inside your body.

The physical brings us home to the temple that is our body; the physical is an embodied sense that steers us home to our physical selves and allows us to touch much, much more.

This may seem straightforward enough. The problem is, however, that many of us have forgotten how to feel. Put this book down for a moment, and reflect:

❭ What do you feel in your body right now?

❭ Get specific. What do your toes feel like?

❭ What does your right thigh feel like?

❭ Get edgy: What does your perineum feel like?

❭ Examples of physical sensations are tingly, warm, solid. (Examples of imagined sensations are golden, shimmery, joy.)

....

....

❭ If you came up with an imagined sensation, try to go deeper.

....

....

❭ Wiggle your toes. What do you feel?

....

....

❭ Rub your thigh with your right hand. What do you feel?

....

....

❭ Find some privacy, and touch your perineum. What does that feel like?

....

....

❭ How is the quality of feeling different from what you experienced the first time?

....

....

If you skip over or merely think about these exercises, you miss the first step.

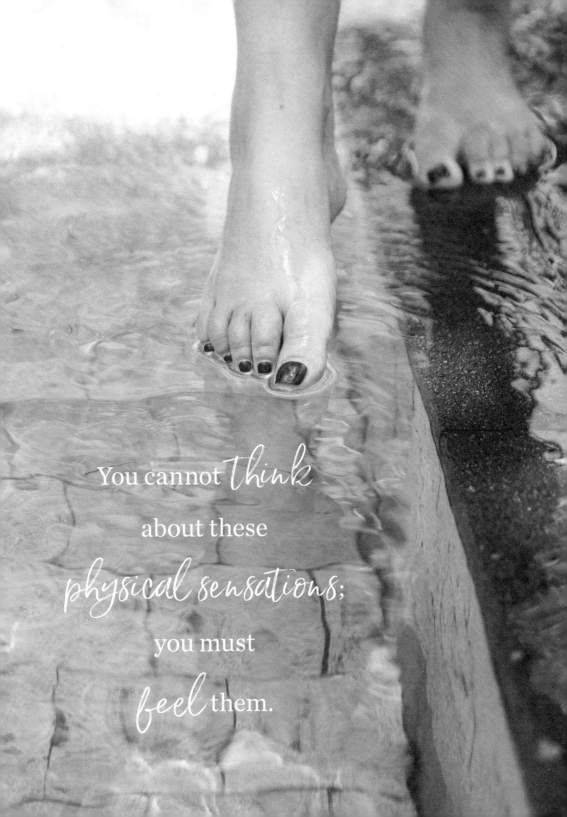

You cannot *think* about these *physical sensations;* you must *feel* them.

Many of us, when we start to tune into our physical sensations (when there is no pain), realize that we do not feel anything at all.

This is not uncommon, as many of us will subconsciously do anything that we can to numb the feelings going on in our body. Many of us are trained from a young age to disassociate from feelings and emotions, like the contraction in the chest, which may accompany fear; eventually, the numbing becomes habitual.

And, in some respects, life is easier this way. A numb life does not have the exuberance and the limitless potential, or the high that can accompany an opening heart; but it also does not have the same level of exposure. A life cannot be lived in Technicolor without the opening of the heart; this in turn will expose our frailties, our wounds, and our vulnerabilities, allowing them to be gently dissolved. When we are experiencing that tender openness, it feels that we can be hurt much more easily. In truth, this is a life lived in courage, for magic emerges once we let go of the fear that keeps us from *not* feeling.

The way to come back into the body is to start to feel.

The way to come back into the body is to start to feel. This takes practice. The pivotal aspect is to start: your ability to feel will grow in time, as you remain committed to the practice.

In Lunar Abundance, the Moon represents the feelings, among other things. It is fundamental to the practice to anchor in our bodies in order to feel the physical sensations; anchoring within is the focal point for the first lunar phase. The New Moon is the time to practice this foundational concept of the Lunar Abundance practice: reconnecting with our bodies.

NASSIM

Nassim is a beautiful woman. She glows with an inner radiance, a kindness that shines from her heart and cannot be cosmetically approximated.

Born in Lisbon, Portugal, to Indian parents, Nassim moved to London, England, when she was seventeen. Nassim loved school and had a supportive family. But as a young girl, Nassim did not feel confident in her body. She did not fit the culturally desired image of a young woman, either for herself or her family; her genetics did not lend themselves to the skinny women who graced the covers of the European magazines. She never learned to swim—routinely teased by her peers, she was never confident enough to wear a swimsuit at the beach near her home. Nassim's relationship with her body was not a deficiency that she created for herself: it was the by-product of a culture that tells us that we need to look a certain way in order to be beautiful. As Naomi Wolf sketches out in the 1990 classic *The Beauty Myth*, the beauty industry needs to fan the flames of low self-esteem in order to sell more products, in turn sustaining itself.

However, identifying the genesis of the problem as external to us does not mean that we are precluded from taking action to change the status quo: it is possible for us to attend to issues that are not of our making. For example, when I was learning to ride a scooter, this was the takeaway message—cars *won't* see you, they *will* put you in danger, it is *not* your fault—and yet you *still* have the power to change the course and end up just fine.

When Nassim was a young girl, she found a way to navigate confusion, discomfort, and aloneness. Bathed at night in moonlight, she would speak to the Moon. She would have a conversation with the Moon. She found that conversation gave her a sense of peace; she felt seen, and she felt understood.

This felt so natural to Nassim, but she had no idea if this was normal. Talking to the Moon, after all, sounds a little odd. Intuitively, she knew that she would be mocked if she mentioned it, so she kept it quiet. It was only much later, in her early thirties, at a time of transition in her life, that she started to reconnect with the Moon. She started to make the link between the Moon phase and how she was feeling in her own body, beginning to uncover deeper resistance to fully

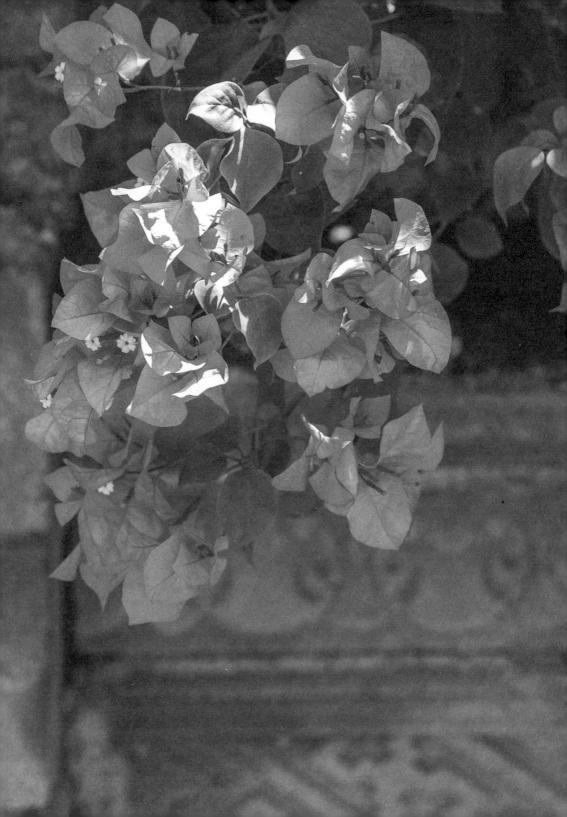

Identifying the genesis
of the problem as *external*
to us does not mean
that we are *precluded* from
taking action to *change*
the status quo:
it is *possible* for us to
attend to issues that are
not of our making.

inhabiting the temple of her own self. She started to return to her feelings. As a woman in her early thirties, searching now for answers of a different kind, she started to remember her nightly conversations with La Luna.

As she feels called to reconnect to the Moon as a woman finding her way in a rapidly changing world, Nassim has started to recognize who she really is, the beauty of her body, and the ability to feel and to move and to dance with joy and abandon, rather than shame. The Moon redirects Nassim's attention back to how she feels in her body, rather than to how she thinks she should look. Starting to feel her body for the first time, Nassim nourishes her body with healthy food that feels good for her. Finally, she realizes that the habitual guilt that she is used to feeling after she eats has fallen away, even without trying. She is attending to her subconscious longing, rather than feeding it with anxiety and fear—external feelings of not being enough.

NEW MOON CEREMONY

The way that Nassim starts to come back to her body—how she starts to feel again—is through her monthly New Moon ceremonies.

The New Moon time and date is in her calendar, so Nassim makes sure in advance that she will not be disturbed for about half an hour that evening. Nassim is a lover of beauty, so she makes her environment beautiful. She loves roses, lilies, and orchids, and adds a few wildflowers plucked from her garden. Fairy lights in her bedroom add some sparkle on a cool autumn evening, and her surplus of sheepskins makes even the English night cozy. Under the skylight to her right sits Nassim's altar, with a statue of Ganesha—the remover of obstacles—rose quartz, amethyst, malachite, rhodonite, and Moonstone, together with Gaya cards. Nassim is in her element in creating comfort, and she lights her rose and lavender candles, tops up her pot of rooibos vanilla tea with coconut milk, and lines up her playlist with Tina Malia, Peia, and Deva Premal.

With all her senses engaged, Nassim finds it easier to close her eyes and become present to what is going on inside: both her emotions and her physical feelings.

Nassim sits and holds her hands together until she starts to feel warmth emerge. She may rub her hands to evoke a greater tingly sensation.

She allows herself to feel whatever comes up, noticing too the urge of wanting to rush to some diagnosis or find the meaning of physical sensations: a burning in her belly, a heaviness in her right leg, a tightness in her lower back.

Nassim just allows herself to feel whatever is physically emerging in her body.

Emotions might also rise. Sadness might well up, and rather than trying to quash it, she feels and experiences it. After a time, Nassim stands and starts to sway to the music, moving her hips in rhythmic motion, allowing whatever is happening to flow through her.

Nassim spends about fifteen or twenty minutes connecting with herself in this way. She doesn't set a timer—the exact time is less important than the experience.

There is just the opportunity to feel. How often do we give ourselves that permission? This is the first part of the practice.

Free lunar journaling resources available for download at www.lunarabundance.com

With her journal next to her, Nassim opens her eyes and documents what she felt where in her body. She also writes down anything else that came up for her.

There is no explicit objective for this New Moon Ceremony, no end point.

There is just the opportunity to feel.

How often do we give ourselves that permission?

This is the first part of the practice.

YOUR NEW MOON CEREMONY

It is time now for you to craft your own New Moon intention-setting ceremony.

It does not need to have all the bells and whistles of Nassim's—mine is not quite so luxe. Or it might have other subtle differences; you might want to introduce cleansing sage or incense, essential oils and upbeat tunes. You might set your intention in the bath or in bed, or you might draw together a posse of women in order to set intentions together. You can see a checklist below to help you craft your own New Moon Ceremony.

The point is to create a situation that feels lush and gorgeous for you.

NEW MOON CEREMONY CHECKLIST

) Work out when you will conduct your New Moon Ceremony. You can check the next New Moon date on the free planner available on my website: www.lunarabundance.com.

) Get specific—write down a date and time, and put a reminder in your calendar now, for 15–30 minutes at least. You may wish to sit at night. Sit as close to the New Moon time as possible, but you don't need to be rigid about the timing.

) Work out where you will be, where you won't be disturbed.

) If you need to ask someone to take care of the kids, or ask your partner or housemates to give you space, make arrangements for this.

) Give some thought as to how to make your space beautiful and comfortable.

+ *Music* (soothing meditation or something a bit more vibrant?)

+ *Taste* (e.g., herbal tea, or, of course, chocolate)

+ *Smell* (e.g., candles, incense, oil, sage)

+ *Visuals* (e.g., flowers, crystals, meaningful trinkets)

+ *Touch* (e.g., fabrics, textiles, any of the above)

Invite your girlfriends to join you

(being by yourself is also okay)

Get your *journal* and *pen* at the ready to jot down any
visions, feelings, thoughts, reflections,
and/or *realizations* that emerge.

Throughout the remainder of the Moon cycle, Nassim continues to feel.

Each night, she looks up at the Moon. She starts to thaw, and in the thaw, she starts to remember who she really is.

And then she starts to wonder—what kind of life might she be able to lead?

SETTING INTENTIONS

Creating a better life starts with being intentional about the life that you want to create. To be clear: it *starts* here, but there is more to travel. In future Moon phases we focus on taking more focused, external action; in this dark Moon phase, the action that we take is to *hone our sense of direction, and set an intention.*

The Moon represents the feelings, so here we focus on how we want to feel. Feeling what we want to feel *now* will help guide us toward intentionally crafting the life that we want to lead. In fact, it can be incredibly helpful to speed up the journey, to close the gap between where we are now and where we want to be.

WHY SET INTENTIONS AT THE NEW MOON?

In a state of constant movement and change, the Moon offers us the potential for change. The Moon has long been associated with fertility, creation, planting, and nourishing and nurturing seeds. The relationship with the Moon and agriculture goes way back, and many cultures garden by the Moon today.[27] Here we find the genesis of the notion of aligning with the Moon cycle for creative purposes—the idea of growing a seed planted in fertile soil speaks eloquently to our capacity for growth and creativity.

Of course, you can set intentions whenever you like. In this lunar practice, we set intentions at the New Moon, seeding them at the first phase in the cycle to harvest them later in the cycle at the Full Moon, or in future Moon cycles (depending on your intention, and what action you take to bring this into form).

WHAT INTENTION SHOULD YOU SET?

The first thing that women often wonder is: What intention should I set? My response is this: What is your dream life, and where is that falling short of your current reality? What strikes me most when I ask this of women is that often the answer is: Oh . . . I hadn't thought about that.

Then it starts to emerge—the knowing, the hope that life can be better.

Oftentimes, when women dare to dream, it is the first time that we step outside what we have been told to think, to do, and to believe. We start to uncover our own desires.

We might be surprised by what we actually want when we give ourselves the space and time to dream. We might be shocked by how bold some of our needs are, or how minimalist. We might also feel uncomfortable with how we feel when we articulate our desires—all totally normal. It is when we start to dream that we start to recognize who we really are, and what we have to give.

Remember that this is a dreaming. We want our hearts to expand in wonderment and possibility; we can ground our hearts in reality later.

Take a moment to pull out a pen and start your dreaming. Do this now—don't skip over the exercise and say you will return to it later.

What is your dream life?

A waking dream, that is.

Take the time to journal here (don't rush, and know there is no right or wrong):

〉 Where do you live?

〉 Are you with a soul mate?

❱ What is your relationship like with your family?

❱ What does your community look like?

❱ Who else is in your life?

❱ What do you do for work?

❱ What is in your bank account?

❱ How are you moving your body?

❱ What are you eating?

❱ How are you giving back?

) Do you have a spiritual practice?

....

....

) What are your self-care practices?

....

....

) What are your hobbies?

....

....

) What are your creative pursuits?

....

....

) How do you feel in your body?

....

....

GIVE YOURSELF THE TIME TO DREAM

It takes courage to dream—to vocalize or write down your desires for your life. It might also take time. It might bring up some "stuff"—guilt, fear, and repressed emotion. Journal about these as well. Remember: we are working here with the Moon as a mirror—if you go through this process, you will start to see your own beliefs about what is and is not possible for your life; and what you do and don't deserve. Pay attention.

Will your dream life come into form? You will need to work with all the phases throughout the Moon cycle to help bring your intentions into form, and we will be working with these phases throughout the rest of the book. Ushering your

Free abundant life audio available at
www.lunarabundance.com

intentions into reality will require effort, and it may take time. How much time will depend on what your wishes are, how distant from your current reality your dream life is, and what you are prepared and able to do to help usher your intention into being, both in this and in subsequent Moon cycles.

The thing is, though, without gaining clarity about what you want, you'll be lurching around without a map. If you want to consciously co-create your life, gaining clarity about what it looks like (and, also important, feels like) is the first step that we are engaged with now.

Allow yourself to feel into all elements of your dream life, and let that clarity crystallize.

INTENTION-SETTING

Return to the above and make notes—where are you currently living your dream life, and where does your life fall short?

Remember, we are not just using "abundance" as another word for "money" in this practice. We want to cultivate a sense of living in the flow; all kinds of abundance in all kinds of areas are relevant, whether that be an abundance of romance, creativity, friends, clients, love, money, luck, fun, travel, offers, peace, or energy.

Review the dream life that you outlined above. Do you have more gaps than expected, or are you already well on the way to experiencing your dream life?

❭ Write out specific gaps between your dream life and current reality.

Turn these gaps around into possible future intentions (frame these in the positive). For example, rather than set an intention based on releasing fear that accompanies your dream to leave the city for a sea change, set an intention based on how you'd feel when you are living by the ocean in a supportive community.

My suggestion is to work with one intention per Moon cycle. Why? Because you will actually be doing things throughout the Moon cycle, and you do not want to get overwhelmed or abandon the practice if you have several intentions at play. I encourage you to pick one intention and return to the others later.

Remember that the Moon cycle is *abundant*. There is always another Moon cycle coming; there are further opportunities to attend to our wishes and desires.

Doing this practice helps you set the scene for how you can start to create a better life for *you*. It helps you to focus your attention right away by selecting an area in which to focus your attention, via intention, at the upcoming Moon cycle.

EXAMPLES OF INTENTIONS

Focus on what your intention *feels* like. Now, intentions are different from goals. In this practice, intentions are thematic and feeling-based. These are thematic, embodied, and felt, rather than specific and objectively measureable.
Goals are also important, but are a bit different from intentions.

Again, you can work with both—in fact, it is potent to work with both.

However, my experience is that we have a surplus of goal-setting advice. Setting intentions in the Lunar Abundance practice takes a different approach; it is the Yin to the Yang of goal-setting. It involves moving beyond the head into physical sensation.

Set both an intention and a goal, if you like. Some intentions may have a corresponding goal; some intentions may focus on qualities, and won't have a goal to match.

An example of an *intention* that has to do with a *quality* (relating):

I feel my *heart opening* as I connect with my *sisters*.

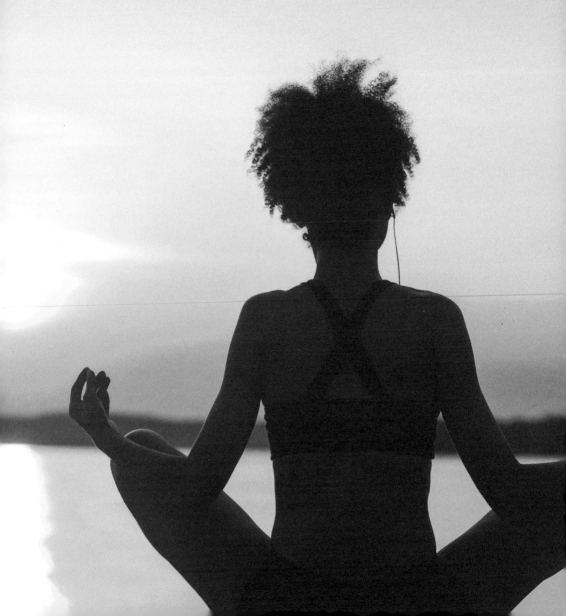

An example of an *intention* with a *corresponding goal* (money):

I feel stable and *grounded* with my

feet on the Earth as I feel a steady flow

of *prosperity* through my life.

The goal: I make $10,000 on top of my current salary in the next 12 months (e.g., through negotiating a pay increase, finding a better-paid job, coaching clients on the side, or selling my old clothes and jewelry online—or a combination of the above)!

Write down your intention for this Moon cycle.

Free intention-declaring resources available for download at www.lunarabundance.com

WHAT IS YOUR INTENTION FOR THIS MOON CYCLE?

Whether you feel it in your hips or heart or somewhere else entirely, put words around your intention now.

While you are feeling your intention, I suggest that you write it down in order to ground the feeling. You can then work with these words to trigger the feeling of your intention, which you can return to every day throughout the monthly cycle. Feeling your intention each morning, even before getting out of bed, is a good place to start; you could also try feeling it in your morning shower, after you have brushed your teeth of an evening, or even in the bathroom at lunchtime. You could add it to an existing daily practice so you remember to do it, each day.

INTENTION-SETTING CEREMONY

If you are new to working with the Moon, you may wish to spend your first New Moon just in a feeling ceremony. You could also carry on your intention-setting process after an intention-setting ceremony.

Feel the physical sensations in your body.

If this is your first time setting an intention, you may wish to review the above list with the gaps between where you currently are in life and where you would like to be.

By tuning into your feelings, direct your attention to the part of your body that feels warm and tingly.

You may want to bow your head to your heart and simply ask the question, "What is my intention?"

Or you may wish to dance.

Or you may wish to go on a walk or a swim.

You may wish to ask for inspiration, pull a book from a shelf, and open it at random to see what leaps out.

Or you may wish to even set an intention to know your intention!

 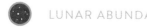

Do not *worry* if your intention
does not arrive.

Ask yourself for *clarity,*
and *be open* to your intention
dropping in whenever
you are *ready*—it often comes
at night, in your *dreams,*
or when you are driving home.

WHEN TO SET AN INTENTION?

Usually I suggest that you set your New Moon intention at the time of the New Moon, or once the new cycle has actually started (in other words, not before the New Moon).

Why? So often we race forward to the Next Thing, without pausing to take stock of where we are. Part of this practice is to reflect on what has come to pass. As the Moon wanes to darkness in the sky, one lunar cycle is drawing to a close. This is the time to take the opportunity to practice reflecting on that previous lunar cycle (you can read more about that later in this book, in the Balsamic Moon phase).

Too often, we don't take the time to look back to celebrate our achievements, or to feel into the best way forward for our dreams. This is why I suggest that we complete one lunar cycle before we start the next. Notice where you have been, give thanks for what you have received or learned, and celebrate!

Then, I suggest that you set your intention on or just after the New Moon. Again, don't worry if it's not on the buzzer. It does not need to be to the minute.

If the New Moon is at 3 a.m., for instance, I don't get up to set my intention. I am busy worshipping at the Temple of Sleep, and I'll set my intention when I awake in the morning.

Remember, in Lunar Abundance we are working with the Moon as a natural timekeeper. We are not suggesting that the Moon is actually making us do something. However, when you set your intention as close to the New Moon as possible, you get the benefit of a full lunar cycle (the month ahead) in which to work with your intention.

The times for different time zones are in my e-letters (and yes, the Moon phases happen at the same time around the world; the phase times are dependent on the Moon's relationship with the orbits of the Sun and Earth).

Are you really feeling it, or just thinking about feeling it? A reminder that when I talk about feelings, I'm talking about *physical sensations*.

Golden is not a physical sensation—it is a (beautiful and inspiring) concept. Your solar plexus is an energetic point, not an organ.

 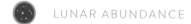

Lunar Abundance is designed to guide you home to your *body*.

If you are feeling physical sensations in your head, say that. If you are feeling jittery in your stomach, say that. Learn to focus on what you actually feel.

What is your intention?

Return to your intention now. Is it the same as it was? If different, write it down again.

❭ What did you learn about yourself in this process?

_____

_____

_____

_____

_____

_____

❭ What might you do differently next time?

_____

_____

_____

_____

_____

_____

❭ How will you make your intention relevant to your daily life throughout the Moon cycle? (e.g., printing it out, writing it out?)

....

....

....

....

....

....

❭ If you plan to sit with the intention each day throughout the cycle, when?

....

....

....

....

....

....

Be realistic, and be kind to yourself. We want to set you up for success by establishing a strong foundation for the rest of the Moon cycle.

This practice is only just beginning.

Summary

> The darkness at the New Moon is an invitation to begin our journey to the well of wisdom. Engage your senses—touch, hearing, smell, taste, and sight—to navigate this process.

> The way to come back into the body is to start to feel. This takes practice. In Lunar Abundance, feelings are physical sensations. Step toward these sensations to steer yourself home toward your physical self. You cannot think about physical sensations: you must feel them.

> Consider creating a New Moon Ceremony in a way that feels luxe, lush, and good for you (refer to the checklist in this chapter for a guide).

> Intentions are set at the New Moon phase. Be realistic and kind to yourself when setting your intention in this first Moon phase, so that you may establish a strong foundation for the rest of the Moon cycle.

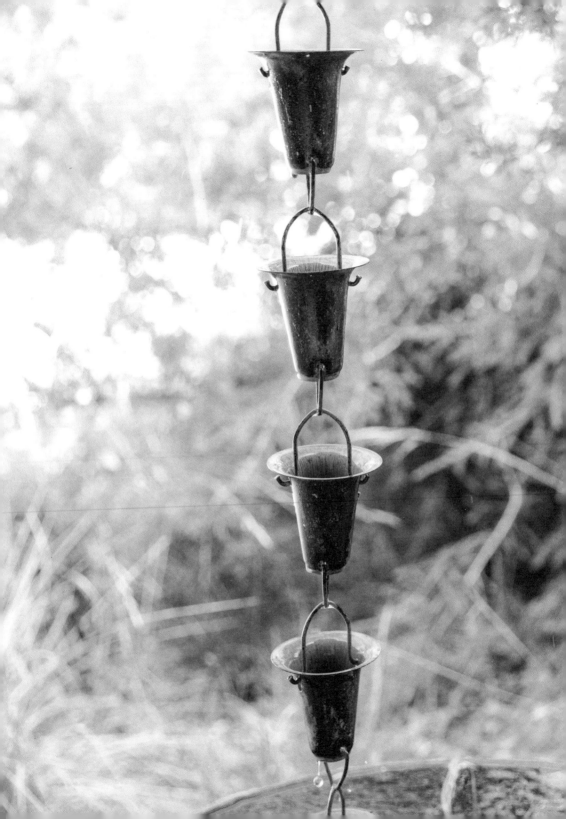

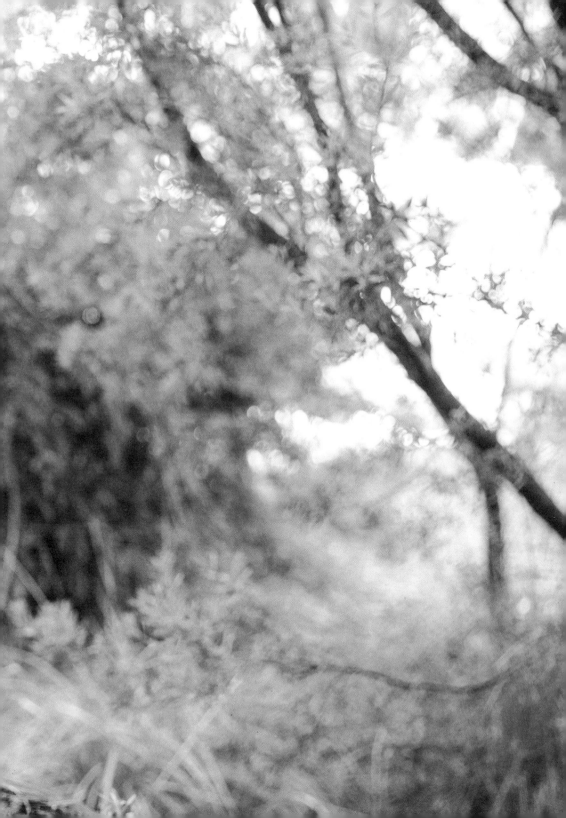

Sometimes the most important
thing in a whole day
is the rest that we take between
two deep breaths . . .[28]

—ETTY HILLESUM

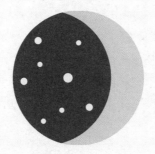

Crescent Moon

A few days after the New Moon, we start to see some light in the sky as the Moon starts to emerge into a crescent shape.

The Moon cycle itself takes around 29 and a half days. This is a little more than the time taken for the Moon to complete a full lap of the Earth; but the Earth also moves around the Sun during that time, so we have just over 29 days to move from one New Moon to the next.

When I started tracking the Moon cycle, I started to feel into every day within the cycle. I now work with the eight phases of the Moon, a method popularized by Dane Rudhyar in his 1960s classic, *The Lunation Cycle*. Why? There's a multitude of ways to divvy up the Moon cycle, after all. In *Moon Phases: A Symbolic Key*, Martin Goldsmith writes of the 28-phase Moon cycle; many others are concerned with the four-phase cycle, or even just the waxing and waning phase cycles. After some experimentation, the eight phases were what made sense to me, as Steven Forrest describes in *The Book of the Moon*: not too long and not too short. In sum, it seemed to offer a method that was meaningful in my very human life.

Setting intentions at the New Moon and then just *waiting* for the next New Moon takes up substantial time—what happens between setting those intentions? Twiddling the thumbs, or nudging issues under the carpet?

Over the course of the Moon cycle, the Moon will wax from New to Full—taking around two weeks—and then from Full back to New—again, roughly two weeks. You may hear that the time when the Moon waxes is the Yang time, the two weeks to initiate projects, and the time when the Moon is waning is the time to take your foot off the gas, or the Yin time. That may indeed be true for you, but what I have found is that merely working with the waxing and waning aspects of the Moon cycle does not make practical sense in terms of my day-to-day life. While developing my Moon practice, I needed more detail than a cycle that merely took one month, or a cycle that was Yang for two weeks, then Yin for two.

On the other hand, checking in on the Moon *every* day did not seem to give the right structure, either. The Moon changes daily; therefore, checking in each day was helpful for me as a cue to check in with how I was feeling that day, but as I started to work with the Moon cycle to bring my intentions to life, daily checking started to border on obsession: Where was the Moon *right now*, and how was I feeling *right now*? I am most interested in patterns, and the daily movement of the Moon did not give me enough to work with on this score. This is why I began to work with the eight Moon phases.

While doing so, I stumbled across the lunar calendars by Sandra and David Mosley, who suggested that the eight Moon phases alternated between Yin and Yang. These would occur in pairs: the New Moon is Yang, and the next in the cycle, the Crescent Moon, is Yin. This concept was presented simply: the notion of having a time to move forward, and a time to restore. It was a moment for me, and I started to play with the Yin and Yang phases of the Moon.

Crescent is the first Yin phase.

The Yin phases show us how to start practicing a better way of living and working. As you shall see, the Yin phases are not about having half the week for leisure, because that does not accurately reflect most lives. We live in the real world, with its plentiful responsibilities. We may be stressed and tired at work because work is stressful and tiring; we are working longer and harder. Changing the game may require us to collectively push back on the cultural mores about workloads, seeking better ways of living and working in the process.

To be clear, my lunar practice does not promise to solve structural issues like *why* the working world is becoming increasingly stressful, or why many women still tend to carry a double load at the office and home. What I aim to do in this book is to cast light on our habitual patterns so that we can locate and exercise the power that we do have, while being clear about the limitations of individual action. As we grow our awareness about what drives us, we can start to unwind the shadow patterns within ourselves and determine which choices we are able to make about how we live our lives—and what might be the domain of bigger projects, beyond the domain of personal choice.

HOW IT WORKS

Within the lunar cycle, we work with eight Moon phases. Four of these are Yin, and four are Yang.

YANG MOON PHASES	YIN MOON PHASES
New Moon	Crescent Moon
First Quarter Moon	Gibbous Moon
Full Moon	Disseminating Moon
Third Quarter Moon	Balsamic Moon

These come in **pairs**, in a polarity that jives with each other. There are four pairs within the Moon cycle: the first part of the pair is Yang, and the second part is Yin. The Moon cycle starts at the New Moon, which is a Yang phase. It makes sense for the cycle to start as Yang, as Yang has the quality of initiation. So the New Moon is the first Yang of the Moon cycle; it is also the first half of the first pair, so it is the Yang of this pair. The second half of the first pair is the Crescent Moon, which is Yin. And then we return to Yang to start the next pair: the First Quarter Moon is Yang, and so on and so forth.

	PAIRS
1	New Moon (Yang), Crescent Moon (Yin)
2	First Quarter Moon (Yang), Gibbous Moon (Yin)
3	Full Moon (Yang), Disseminating Moon (Yin)
4	Third Quarter Moon (Yang), Balsamic Moon (Yin)

So the Crescent Moon phase, the phase in which we currently find ourselves, is the first of the Yin phases.

YIN AND YANG: RELATIVE TERMS

The Yin and Yang phases are not just interesting ideas—these provide the framework for a way of *living*. Most of what I learned about Yin and Yang I learned from Kevin Farrow, who has been influenced by Taoism, Qi Gong, and other traditions.[29]

Think back to the classic Yin/Yang symbol. There is Yin in the Yang and Yang in the Yin: a black dot in the white, a white dot in the black. So there will also be

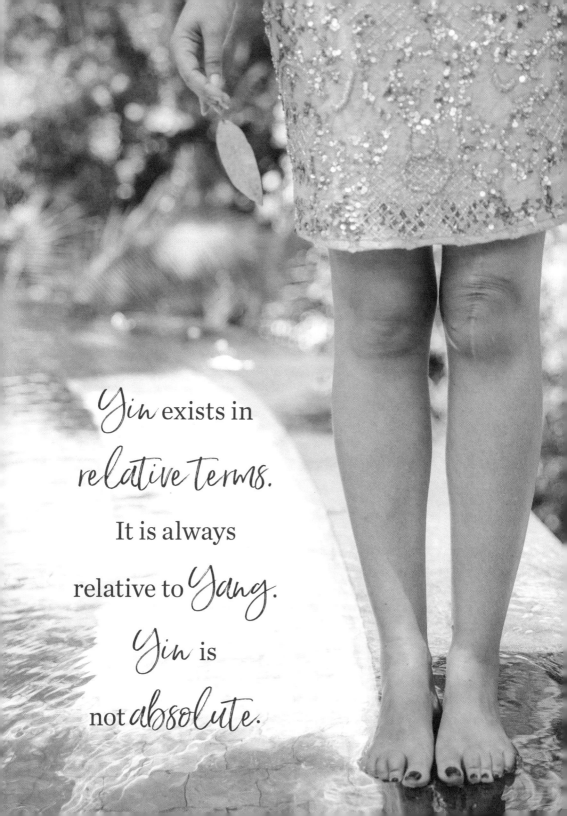

Yin exists in *relative terms.* It is always relative to *Yang. Yin* is not *absolute.*

part of the Yin in your Yang, and part of the Yang in your Yin. What this means is that there will be points of action and moving forward in your Yin phase, and there will also be rest in your Yang phase.

Again—it is all relative, and the polarity is key. Some characteristics of Yin and Yang:

YANG	YIN
Doing	Being
Initiating	Restoring
Speaking	Listening
Giving	Receiving

Some things are not about Yang or Yin at all: presence, intelligence, wisdom, and embodiment transcend Yang and Yin. In the ways in which I work with them, Yang and Yin are modes of operating. We all need Yang and Yin to operate effectively. You can be a woman and identify, in general, as more Yang. You can be a man and identify, in general, as more Yin. Regardless of gender, you can be Yang at work and Yin with your lover. You can be Yin with one lover and Yang with another; Yin during the entrée when dining out with a friend, and Yang with the same friend over dessert. You might be Yang at work, and Yin in your physical fitness routine. You might be Yang in some aspects of your work, and Yin in other respects.

Relativity is the key point. In the application of this lunar practice, your Yin Moon phase will look different from my Yin phase. One of your Yin phases may be different from another of your Yin phases. The Balsamic Moon phase—which is a Yin phase that we shall explore later in this book—may make the Crescent Moon phase look Yang. Your Yin phases will look different from your Yang phases. Your Crescent Moon phase will look different from your First Quarter Moon phase.

There is nothing wrong with any of this, by the way. Yin and Yang are neutral; neither is good or bad. What might become ineffective is when you lose your own sense of harmony between the two modes and rely on one over the other.

What that harmony looks like will be particular to you, and elucidating this particular makeup is essential for you to find your flow. This is what you will find through working with the Moon cycle in the exercises throughout this book. Practice is necessary to garner actual experience of this harmony, which in turn will help you understand how this looks in your own life, as well as what your natural rhythms and optimum flow may be.

I use these terms as a kind of therapeutic metaphor: to demonstrate concepts and invite practical application, rather than to suggest that the Moon and Sun are trying to make you do anything or be a particular way. In Lunar Abundance, we work with the Moon as "Yin" and the Sun as "Yang." This means that the monthly lunar cycle is Yin, as compared to the annual Yang cycle of the Sun. There are too many cultural differences to say that this is the way that the Moon and Sun objectively *are*—it is just the way that makes sense for me. For example, the Incas had a Moon goddess, Mama Killa, and a Sun god, Inti, but Candi and Chandra are the Hindu Moon god and goddess who take turns at representing the Moon each month.[30]

Regardless of who's who, we do often find a male/female personification in those representing the Moon and the Sun. Cultures with Moon gods usually have a Sun goddess—the almighty Egyptian Isis scored both, but more frequently we find a polarity, such as the Nordic Mani (Moon god) and Sol (Sun goddess) or the Australian Aboriginal Warlpiri Sun woman and Moon man. The polarity point is often played out with eclipses, the point at which the Sun and Moon's two orbits intersect with the lunar nodes. For the Warlpiri, when the Moon caught up with the Sun, this was a time of lovemaking.[31]

It is this sense of lovemaking and creative sizzle that has an allure for me, and this is what I play with in Lunar Abundance: the polarity between the Sun and the Moon, as well as within the Yin and the Yang phases of the Moon cycle.

We dive deeper into creative flow in the next chapter on a Yin phase, Gibbous Moon. For the moment, I note that out of all the concepts that I now share, the concept of Yin is the one that has challenged my clients the most. Your first question may be: Yes, yes, very nice, but what do we do in a Yin phase? How can I run a company, have a baby, get promoted, work out, meditate every day, eat properly, be a good friend (wife, daughter, mother, sister, boss, cat lover), and/or start that side business—*and* be Yin?

We live in a world where the qualities of doing and hustling are celebrated, to such a degree that the concept of "being" has been devalued. The reality is that this impacts both our quality of life and our effectiveness. Bringing back the Yin is not only more conducive to your well-being: it is also the path to sustainable success.

But you do not need to opt out of the mainstream system to work with the Yin phases. Running my own show has also been a way to stop indulging the cultural proclivity for overwork, because I can set my own hours—I still work hard, but on my own terms, and I also have fun. But entrepreneurship is not for everyone, and what the purveyors of "the dream" rarely share is that building a business from scratch requires a great deal of time and effort. There are ways to incorporate the Yin phases into an employee work life; I know because I have done so, and will share ways that may make sense for you.

Are your Yin or Yang qualities underdeveloped?

Also—it is not all just about work! Yang and Yin are not just about work/life balance, where Yang is work and Yin is life, with an aim to find an equilibrium somewhere in the middle. As anyone with small children can attest, going to the office can feel like a mini-vacation! Work/life balance is an elusive concept, which has been too slippery for me to make meaningful in my own life. Rather, the Yin phases help us with an approach to life *and* work that is more sustainable, and that foregrounds our own self-care so that we can fully enjoy our lives, and in turn help others.

Are your Yin or Yang qualities underdeveloped?

If one of your modes of operating is underdeveloped, the other may become overdeveloped. To be clear, I do not suggest that women "should" be more Yin, or men be more Yang; nor do I think we need a 50/50 split. Your natural and happy disposition may be very, very Yin or very, very Yang.

This question is designed to bring you greater awareness about how you might be operating in various areas of your life; you may be functioning in a way that is normalized in our society, but that may not be serving you. More specifically, I draw attention to how our culture values Yang qualities over Yin, and I hope to shed light on these patterns so you might operate in a way that is most effective for you.

To illustrate: after my fall, I was unable to walk for several months. I was lucky to have a strong right leg to pick up the slack, but over several years my right leg continued to carry the load, eventually overcompensating for my weaker left leg. This was helpful at the time of injury rehabilitation, but over the years it became a pattern that was not productive for the healing of my left leg, nor for the ongoing use of my right leg; the muscles in the left leg started to atrophy as the entire right side of my body progressively tightened, leading to ongoing discomfort as my entire body became out of kilter. Many years later, a bodyworker described my physical dynamic as this: my left leg was an underdeveloped child, and my right leg was an overbearing parent. Its interference in my life was low at first, but when I started to rebalance that unhealthy dynamic, it had a noticeable effect on my physical well-being (and my emotional wellness—the mind and body are interlinked, after all).[32]

It is the health of your own Yin/Yang dynamic that I encourage you to pay attention to, and not the precise breakdown. Your general disposition will guide whether you find the Yin or Yang phases more difficult. The more difficulty you have, the more likely it is that it might be time to pay attention to that area.

You are a complex and multivalent being. For the purposes of this chapter, consider which of the statements on page 95 resonate with you more (as a general rule).

If you fall into the former category, you may be more Yin in nature. If you are most adept at the Yin, or Being, mode, then you will find that the Yang Moon

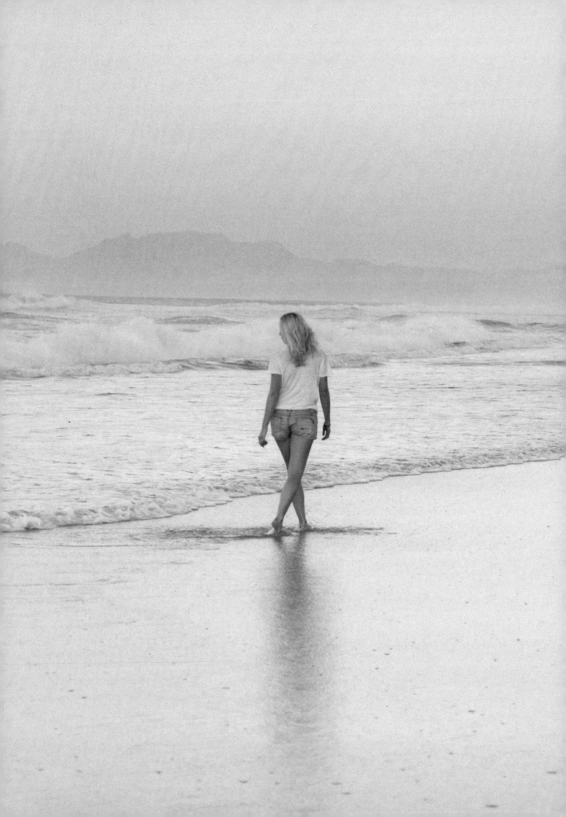

Do you find it difficult to
get *motivated* and initiate *action?*

Or

Are you *tired*, but find it
difficult to *relax*—not because
there are actual things
that you *need to do* to keep
a roof over your head, but
because you are *so wired* that
you cannot "turn off?"

phases may be welcome reminders to get going—in work, yes, but also in other areas of your life, as you will see in the section on holistic living.

On the other hand, if you are in the latter category, you may be more Yang in nature, as I am—at least in my professional life. I would run until my tank was almost empty, and then my body would force me to rest. If you relate to this—to the sense of feeling run-down—then it may be that our cultural disposition toward Yang is not serving you well.

The rest of this chapter is directed toward helping you explore how to cultivate greater harmony through working with the Yin phases of the Moon cycle. Intentional rest is not only essential for our well-being; it also has much to do with our effectiveness.

Where are you more Yin, and where are you more Yang?

The questions below are an opportunity to explore where in your life you notice yourself as being more Yin, and where you are more Yang. Your answers may change over time. Please practice self-compassion with what you find—there are no right or wrong answers, only an opportunity to gain self-knowledge.

> One example: in Lisa's relationship with her employee, Marcos, she tends to be more direct and assertive, telling him what to do and initiating action and projects—so she's often more Yang in that specific professional environment. However, in her relationship with her girlfriend Elspeth, Lisa often finds herself more likely to listen and receive what Elspeth has to offer; she is more Yin.

Consider your own roles in the following situations:

❭ Professional relationship with [e.g., your employee or employer]

❭ Professional relationship with [e.g., your client or supplier]

_____

_____

_____

_____

❭ Professional relationship with [e.g., your colleague or peer]

_____

_____

_____

_____

❭ Family

_____

_____

_____

_____

❭ Intimate relationship with . . .

_____

_____

_____

_____

☽ Friendship with . . .

....

....

....

....

☽ Friendship with . . .

....

....

....

....

☽ Exercise practice

....

....

....

....

☽ Spiritual practice

....

....

....

....

❯ What have you noticed in this exercise?

....

....

....

....

❯ Are you surprised by how Yin you are?

....

....

....

....

❯ Are you surprised by where you are Yang?

....

....

....

....

❯ Do you feel that you have a healthy Yin/Yang dynamic [no wrong answer]?

....

....

....

....

ESSENTIAL: SLOW DOWN

A common fear among high achievers concerns letting go of the Yang overwork and allowing space for Yin. We fear that if we are not striving and working long hours, then we will not be as effective. That is not the case: in fact, slowing down, playing, and experiencing the Yin is where we double our power. Our standard can still be excellence. In fact, our standards can *rise*, with research showing that the mind solves complex problems while in a rest state,[33] and that elite violinists do not play for more hours than average ones, but are instead more focused during the "on" times, relaxing and restoring in the "off" times.[34] Rather than striving to be successful, then, we can rise to excellence without collapsing into a puddle at the end. It is, quite frankly, a more peaceful and enjoyable way to be successful—reaching goals and outcomes without burning yourself out.

In its most extreme manifestation, unhealthy Yang can result in extreme stress. James Doty, a mindful neurosurgeon, explains the concept of fight-or-flight in *Into the Magic Shop*. He writes that when the brain perceives a threat, the part of the autonomic nervous system called the sympathetic nervous system kicks in and releases epinephrine. The hypothalamus releases hormones, triggering the adrenal gland and producing cortisol. This results in narrowing vision, increased heart rate, slowed digestion, and dry mouth. It also results in a suppressed immune system, headaches, and insomnia.[35] Doty writes about how, as a boy in a dysfunctional and highly stressful home setting, he met a woman in a magic shop who taught him how to open his heart and relax, strategies that he draws on today in operations where the stakes are literally life and death. He is able to slow down his breathing, regulate his blood pressure, and be highly responsive.

This is an extreme example of what it means to be out of balance, but it does show that learning to relax during Yin phases is not merely a "nice to have," but is *critical*. If we stay anchored in the go-go-go, the reality is that we will not be as effective. When we have been in "doing" mode at the expense of "being," and we then open up to more of the Yin, the pause allows space for magic. It allows us to create the conditions for abundance; when we are relaxed, our heart opens and we become magnetic.

Extensive research shows that breathing can activate the vagus nerve within the parasympathetic nervous system, and immediately bring us into a deeper state of relaxation.[36] We need both Yin and Yang modes to find homeostasis: a balance. And when we are relaxed, we are more alert and able to notice what is going on around us, and are able to make good choices when presented with them.

Ultimately, tune into your body and do what feels right for you—not what someone else tells you to do. How do you feel in your body at this moment in time? The Yin phases are guides to help you tune into yourself and to practice slowing down; this is not another area where you "should" be a certain way.

Yin phases are the ultimate permission slip to honor your body, to tune in and listen to what she is telling you, and to make decisions accordingly. When you align your self-care with the Moon, you can predict the Yin phases (recall that in this practice we work with the Moon as a natural timekeeper).

The structure of the Yin and Yang phases in the Moon cycle mean that you do not need to have a dialogue with yourself about it being time to relax—you can outsource this to nature, and just pay attention to when the Moon phase shifts into Yin. You can also work with the Yin phases regardless of whether you have a menstrual cycle, although I always encourage you to pay attention to your body first and foremost.

We need both Yin and Yang to find a balance . . .

Many of us do not know what our own rhythms actually are. Squeezed into the five-days-on-and-two-days-off—if not seven days on-on-on—we come to a point where we are often fatigued and not operating as our best selves. We may be operating in a way that is out of balance without even realizing it.

The Yin phases offer a way to come back into connection with ourselves—to understand who we really are, how we feel, what is our ideal pace, and what our bodies desire of us.

This may seem like a revolutionary concept, but it is in accordance with natural rhythms. Tune in and learn your natural ebbs and flows, and then work out practical ways to implement these in your life. You may be surprised at the

Who are you,
really?

What do you
desire?

What do you
need?

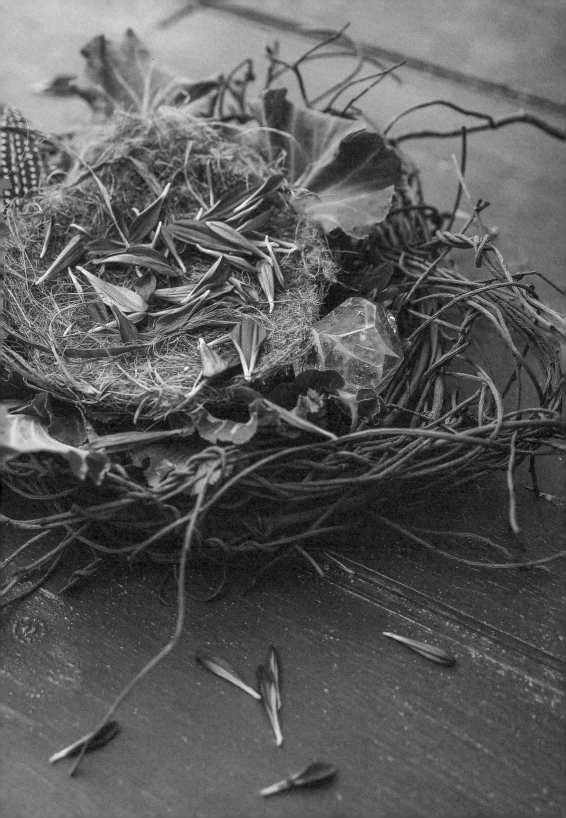

results. Don't forget, too, that the system repeats, meaning that there are more Yin phases ahead, and an abundance of opportunities to keep exploring.

Ask the questions: *Who are you, really?* What do you desire? What do you *need*, on all levels—your mind, body, and heart? Pay attention as this practice reveals the answers to you over time. You will find that layers upon layers are revealed to you as you go deeper, not just in thought, but also in your lived and felt experience.

Summary

❭ This is the first of the Yin phases. The Yin phases are a way to conceptualize downtime and help us navigate a busy schedule. They show us how to start practicing a better way of living and working.

❭ The Lunar Abundance practice works with eight Moon phases alternating, in pairs, between Yin and Yang. Therefore, within the lunar cycle, four phases are Yin and four are Yang. The Crescent Moon is the Yin phase that corresponds to the New Moon.

❭ Yin phases are a guide to help you to tune into yourself and to practice slowing down. These are the ultimate permission slip to tune into your body.

❭ Yin and Yang are relative. What these phases will look like, in practice, will depend on the contours of your own life and work.

❭ It is not only more conducive to your well-being to bring back the Yin; it is a pathway to sustainable success.

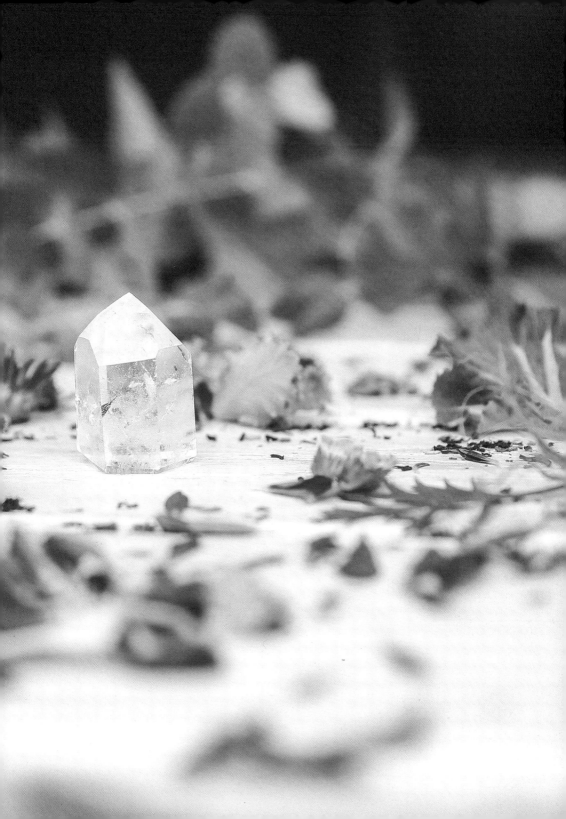

I do not sing because I am happy.
I am happy because I sing.[37]

—DR. WILLIAM JAMES

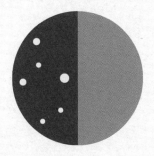

First Quarter Moon

At the First Quarter Moon phase, the Moon appears to be half-full in the sky.

This is the time at which the Moon is midway in its waxing from the darkness of the New to the light of the Full—it is a quarter of the way around the Earth, hence the name for this Moon phase. In this lunar practice, at the First Quarter phase, as the Moon is illuminated in the sky and casts down light upon us, we move into our own illuminated action here on Earth.

In the plant cycle, this is the time associated with putting down roots; in the seasonal cycle, it is a time when spring transitions to summer with the equinox; in the life cycle, our youth is in full swing; in the day's cycle, we hit noon; in our annual cycle, we reach the three-month period after our birthday as we fully settle into our new age and cast our eyes forward to the rest of the year.[38]

This is a Moon phase where we take *action*, taking life into our own hands and shepherding our New Moon intention into tangible form. Up until this point we have been clarifying and feeling our dreams and intentions to inform or illuminate our actions; at the First Quarter Moon phase, we take the right steps to make these dreams come into being.

This is a mindful approach to action, determining and then doing what is most important, à la Greg McKeown's *Essentialism: The Disciplined Pursuit of Less*, rather than merely spinning one's wheels in an addiction to "busy-ness." The essence of this Moon phase is about moving forward—*after* you become clear about where you are going and strategic about your direction, rather than *doing* for the sake of it. "Illuminated action," in the words of spiritual and personal development author Carolyn Myss, is essential to being effective with any desire or project.

It is also time to move once you have a semblance of rest, which we practiced in the previous phase: the Crescent Moon, a Yin phase. We cannot languish in Yin all of the time—unfortunately or fortunately, depending on your perspective! It is through the dance between the doing and the being, the allowing and the initiating, the receiving and the giving that we find our greatest effectiveness in this modern world. In fact, it is in this First Quarter Moon phase that we start to see how we can be more productive once we have gone easy on ourselves for a short time. Consider the arrow—once it has been pulled back, it can fly forward to hit the bull's-eye with speed and precision. We build our muscle and hone our focus over time. We pull back arrow after arrow in our archery practice until we develop the muscle memory and feel it in our body. This is what we practice over and over throughout each Moon cycle, and it is why repetition amplifies this practice.

Experiencing the Yin and Yang phases in practice is the way to alternate modes of being and doing, in a way that is practical and meaningful in your life.

MORE AND LESS EFFECTIVE YANG

Having worked in the law and now in business, I personally know many women and men who predominantly operate in Yang mode and are just fine—who go and go all the time, who love the living daylights out of the doing mode, who are committed irrevocably to their work not as some kind of avoidance strategy, but because they are on a mission to make a positive impact in their chosen area.

These people have their own healthy Yin/Yang dynamic that I mentioned in the previous chapter. If this is you, this chapter is not intended to problematize you—I celebrate you and your mission.

However, if your habitual tendency is to zoom along at a fast clip, and your health/family life/connection to heart and soul suffers; if you draw a blank when someone asks you what your hobbies are; if the last time you remember *What does your Yang look like?* having fun was getting drunk at your best friend's wedding last year; if you ignore the quiet whispers of your heart and distract your shaking hands with deadlines; if you rely on coffee to get through the day and wine to unfurl at night; if you are seeking a better way—then the salient question may be: What is driving you?

In my case, there was an element of identity wrapped up in external achievement. By the time I entered academia, my imposter syndrome was in full bloom, certain that I would soon be recognized as a fraud. The only way that I could see to succeed was to push harder; I was not living in flow at all.

Our addiction to work widens the Cartesian crevasse between our mind and body, between our head and our heart.

What does your Yang look like?

This phase is designed to help women who feel trapped in doing and achieving who *want* to slow down, but do not know *how*. I know many women who have operated in the doing mode for 5, 10, or 20 years—and who seek a better way of living and working, of still being effective and not wearing themselves out in the process.

The action in this lunar phase is not about working or pushing harder, but rather about becoming smarter in the way that we work. Most of those with whom I work tend to operate in a Yang way of being, and feel a sense of disharmony about this. Such disharmony might be because our world values Yang qualities. Given that we often have more difficulty with becoming Yin rather than Yang, the emphasis in this chapter is not on how to become more Yang, but rather, on how to work most effectively with Yang energy.

In this phase, then, as the Moon waxes from New to Full, the focal point is about smart action.

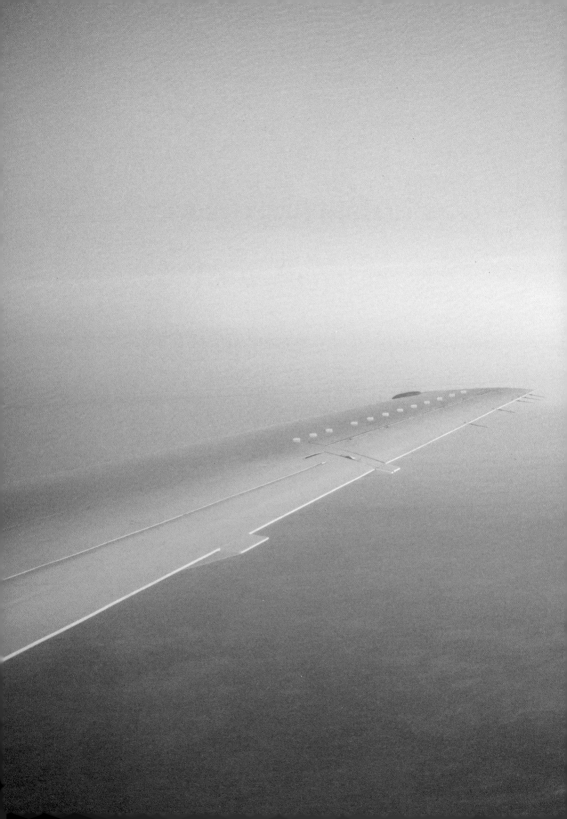

In this phase, then, as the *Moon waxes* from *New* to *Full,* the focal point is about *smart action.*

WAYS THAT YANG CAN BE MORE AND LESS EFFECTIVE

Even when we have balanced our inner Yin and Yang modes, we may play out one or the other more or less effectively. The table below shows ways in which an ineffective Yang may play out, as well as the more fully expressed form.

	LESS EFFECTIVE YANG	EFFECTIVE YANG
Doing... why?	Achievement-oriented	Purpose-driven
Moving... where?	Random busy-ness	Focused direction
Speaking... how?	Overly intellectualized	From head + heart
Giving... how?	Pushy + dominant	Assertive + respectful

Where might you be playing out less effective Yang in your life?

Dr. Paulin Clance first identified "imposter syndrome" in the 1970s during therapeutic sessions with high-achieving women.[39] Symptoms include feeling that your achievements are undeserved, assuming that everyone is smarter or better than you, and a persistent concern that your true inabilities will soon be discovered.[40] Even highly capable sufferers of imposter syndrome are unable to internalize or find a sense of comfort with their own abilities. Imposter syndrome is not gender-specific, but women often catch a more virulent strain. This gives rise to a critique of imposter syndrome as problematizing a lack of confidence, often on the part of women, whereas the issue may more importantly be the *entitlement* of those who are pushy, overbearing, and have a false sense of their own abilities.[41]

Imposter syndrome—and perfectionism—can be significant roadblocks that keep us from taking discerning action (at the other end of the spectrum, entitlement syndrome can have a similar effect).

Do you identify with symptoms of imposter syndrome?

If so, what are concrete ways in which this may affect you in Yang phases?

DISCERNMENT

In ancient Egypt, the principle of Ma'at was that of ethical living, truth, and justice. In her personification as goddess, Ma'at governed the Moon and seasons, the stars and cosmos. She created order among the chaos, which was much needed in the face of society's growing complexity. The individual, the collective, the Earth, Sun, and Moon, the celestial rhythms, the patterns of nature, and the universe: all were organized and understood in equilibrium with the principle and guiding hand of Ma'at. According to her principle, no one should cause pain or sadness to others, harm animals, damage land, hurt waters; these ideals notably link her to aspects of the bigger picture, such as the community and natural environment.[42]

Even the Pharaohs held Ma'at in their heart—she saw below the surface to guide you to act with integrity and discernment. Her blue ostrich feather was her calling card. Once a soul left the mortal body, Ma'at would use the feather to weigh the soul (heart), which then determined whether you had led a life in line with these principles. If so, you were allowed to enter the afterlife; if not, you were condemned to remain in the Underworld.

Ma'at represents the epitome of discernment. Discernment is the ability to make sound judgments and perceive the truth. It involves an understanding of what to cultivate, and what to release or refrain from adopting. As Dr. Mariana Caplan writes, discernment provides individuals with the ability to make "intelligent, balanced and excellent choices in their lives" as "their eyes are wide open, and they see clearly." Importantly, she adds that discernment does not mean that those who possess this skill are immune from failure or mistakes; but, it does enable them to more quickly and carefully turn lapses of judgment into transformative learning experiences.[43]

Jungian analysts Marion Woodman and Elinor Dickson write that "[r]esiding in Ma'at is not a literal undertaking. It means allowing consciousness to move constantly within oneself."[44] The wisdom and integrity of Ma'at infuse our action at this Moon phase. Discernment is about taking conscious action intended to move you closer toward your goals and objectives. What actual action you take at this phase will depend on your own objectives and context. I cannot tell you what your own discerning action should be—in fact, that would defeat the point—but I do hope to guide you toward finding that inner knowing. You don't need to do this all on your own. Nondiscerning action may be acting as a result of the following:

> Out of habit;

> Because we don't think that we are good enough, as in imposter syndrome;

> Because other people want us to act in a certain way, so they tell us to.

It may well be that your habits are serving you; it may be that others have great ideas, and that acting on their advice would serve you.

Or that may not be the case at all.

This is exactly what we are able to unwind if we delve into our subconscious minds, and find more effective ways of operating.

Why do we act in these ways? It is easier—at least in the short term. However, this is exactly what is keeping us stuck in the here and now. It is exactly what is keeping us in the place of low-level irritation—in this place, our life is tolerable enough to carry on, but we remain in a continual state of distraction. It keeps us in the place where we have dreams, but are not getting to where we consciously want to go, which is what we defined at the start of the Moon cycle with our New Moon intention.

Your New Moon intention is your reference point.

Sometimes the most discerning action is inaction: actually saying *no*; finding the spaces where you can exercise agency and exert influence; recognizing that your time is finite. Recognizing where you prioritize your work, but where further work will not actually be helpful, and where you would be better to prioritize your family, health, and friends. Or when it is time to put the pedal to the metal, taking discerning action by determining your priorities and purpose.

Over time, this is something that you will learn; as you grow to know yourself more deeply through this practice, you will fine-tune your intuition and have a sense of how various paths feel in your body. It is also helpful to act and reflect on your actions, instead of just dreaming. Finally, it is essential to draw back and determine your priorities for effective living. In order to prioritize, you need to know what is actually important to you; this requires self-knowledge.

PRIORITIES EXERCISE

How will you know which action to pick at this stage?

Working out which action to pick means returning to the New Moon intention that you've set (this is the point of the bigger intention-setting process in that chapter), and also to work out your priorities in your daily life. Over time, as you gain a better grasp of the contours of how your patterns play out in life, this will become increasingly obvious.

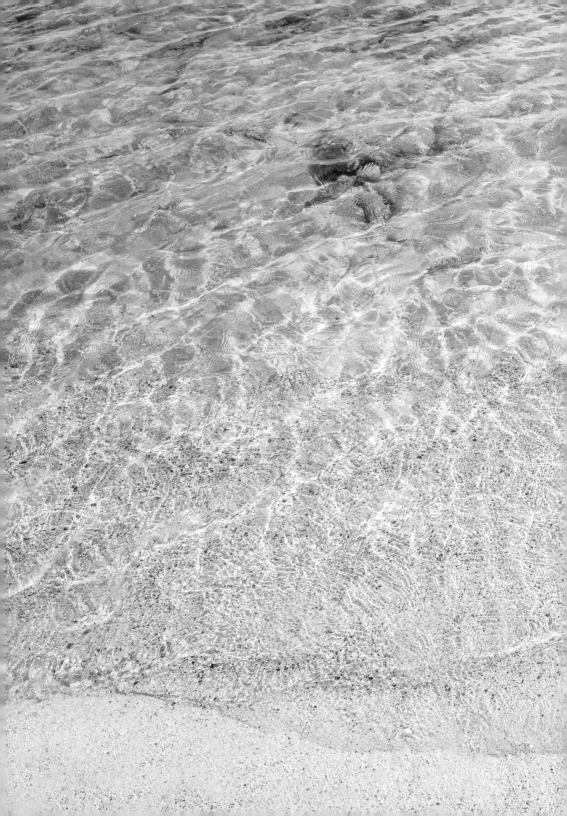

Don't *wait* until things go awry *before* you ascertain what is actually *important to you*.

You don't need to wait until things go awry before you ascertain what is actually important to you. If you are in a slow phase of your life, it might be an ideal time for you to work out your priorities; this will help shape your life for when the inevitable growth phase comes.

And remember—it is not all about work. How can you round out your life and make it more holistic?

DETERMINING YOUR NON-NEGOTIABLES

What are your top priorities—your non-negotiables?

These may include your priorities regarding how you wish to act in the world, toward whom you feel a duty, and what principles you wish to underpin your actions. You could make two lists: one with concrete examples, such as taking care of your children, taking care of your clients, deepening your relationship with your partner, or trying to get a certain number of hours of sleep per night; the second list would contain non-negotiables having to do with qualities that you wish to cultivate, such as kindness to others, and compassion with yourself.

When you are next given the opportunity to act, you can then assess the opportunity against your priorities, rather than giving a knee-jerk yes or no.

❭ Your non-negotiables are (list up to five to eight; don't forget to include yourself)

1. ....

2. ....

3. ....

4. ....

5. ....

6. ....

7. ....

8. ....

Recall your intention. How does that dovetail with your non-negotiables?

If there is not a match, consider whether you could revise either your non-negotiables or your intention.

PURPOSEFUL ACTION

Is there anything on your non-negotiable list that you are not currently still doing?

Why not?

What illuminated action could you take at this Moon phase to make sure that you start following your non-negotiables?

Again, remember that we work with the Moon cycle as a guide. You can take illuminated action at *any* stage, but in Lunar Abundance, it is the First Quarter phase that gives a focal point upon which to practice this principle.

And we are constantly paying attention to our own rhythm—our own ebb and flow. As you follow the exercises in this chapter, you are one step closer to discovering your own rhythm, your own needs, and what makes you tick.

Summary

❯ Illuminated action is important—you *do* need to take action. The most effective action comes after rest, and with discernment.

❯ Working smarter, not harder, helps you to realize your objectives.

❯ Discerning action requires you to get clear on your objectives—and prioritize.

❯ Be courageous in saying no when an action does not fit your greater purpose.

❯ To help you determine what action to take during this phase, refer back to your New Moon intention, and work out your priorities and non-negotiables.

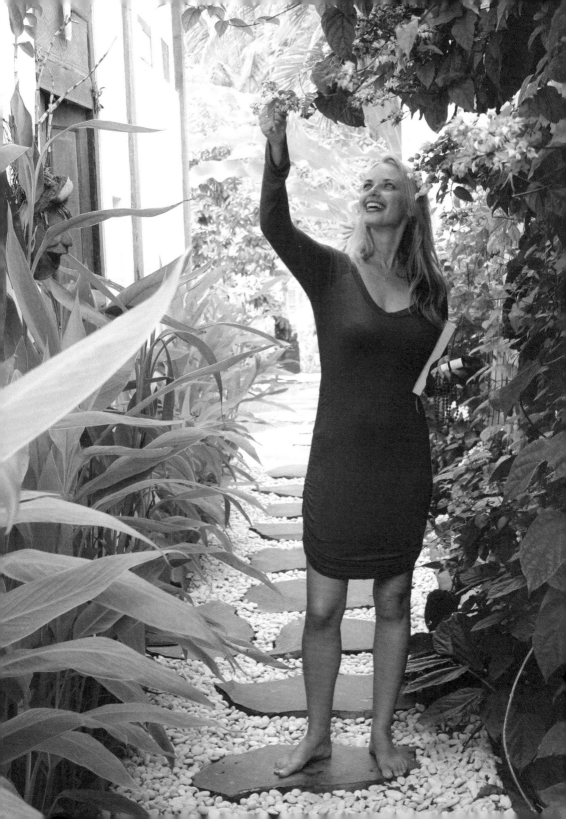

I am not afraid of storms,
for I am learning how to sail my ship.[45]

—LOUISA MAY ALCOTT

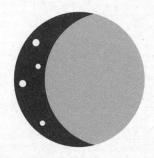

Gibbous Moon

*A couple of years back, I visited San Francisco for a women's con-
ference. On a Tuesday, I had been out sightseeing on foot, catching sight
of a mall while wending my way home.*

Thinking this an opportune moment to stock up on underwear that I had
neglected to pack for the trip, I embarked upon deciphering the American mall
system. While making my way through the belly of the beast—the cosmetics
section of a well-known department store, the type of place that I generally try to
avoid—I was intercepted by a makeup artist for a well-known brand, who, wide-
eyed, whispered urgently, "Oh please, can you do me a favor? Can I give you a
facial? Free? The president of our organization is here, and I really, really do not
want to have to talk to her."

Assuming this was a creative ploy to get me pliantly into a chair to sell me
expensive products, I declined, but she then jerked her head to the nearby
counter—where an imperious, presidential-type, blonde woman *was* standing,
surrounded by a bevy of men and women sternly surveying a display of
moisturizers and grilling another quivering makeup artist.

"Well, why not?" I said.

"Oh my goodness, thank you. You have no idea. Thank you! Thank you so much!"

Let's call our effusive friend Lona.

"No problem. I happen to have a bit of time to spare."

Lona carefully settled me into the makeup chair, beaming as she asked, "Right, so what do you like least about your face?"

What do I like least about my face?

Out loud, "Um, sorry . . . ?"

Subtext: I like my face!

Lona, moderately ruffled, "Oh! I mean—we will start with your eyes—what are you are most worried about? Your dark circles, your lines, or your puffiness?"

I blinked quickly, processing.

Should I be worried about my eyes?

"Oh—I don't know . . ."

Subtext: I am not worried about my eyes . . .

Lona shuffled uncomfortably.

Oh gosh. I am being difficult.

I turned to the mirror to search for flaws.

Well, I guess . . .

"My . . . dark circles?"

"Oh! Great! I can fix those!"

Relieved, Lona fussed with some small bottles and jars.

"Great!" I mirrored—feeling stirred up about how rapidly I fell into faulting my appearance, but also pleased that I got the right answer (tick!) and overcame discord with the otherwise cheerful Lona (tick!).

We both felt better, momentarily.

Lona delved into her deepest drawer and reemerged with a pair of tiny brushes.

"We don't usually use these for store facials, but they are amazing! You'll see!"

At that moment, the perfectly coiffed president swept by with her flock.

"Hello," she greeted me, her lips spreading into a smile, her eyes coolly appraising my outfit and the tiny brushes. "It looks like you are being well cared for here."

Lona deftly switched brushes, keeping her eyes studiously fixed on the cream she was applying to my under-eyes. Her shaking hand was almost imperceptible.

"Oh, yes," I replied. "Lona is taking very good care of me."

Catching sight of myself in the mirror behind the president's group, I couldn't help but notice that I did seem a little disheveled—I had just been walking, I supposed.

"You are—Australian?" asked the president. "How cute!" Her eyes softened.

"Yes. Just visiting San Francisco for a week. I'm here for a conf—"

"We are soon to open our first flagship store in Sydney."

The president exchanged a meaning-laden glance with two of her cronies.

"Oh, well, that's great!" I half-smiled back, feeling the tension. "Maybe I'll, um, visit sometime." I repeated, "Lona really is looking after me well."

The president's smile tightened as she nodded and click-clacked away with the crowd.

Phew.

"Thank you!" whispered a blushing Lona, who was glancing up at me. "So much."

The relief was fleeting.

"Oh, Lona, what's going on?" I cried out, glancing in the mirror again to see an angry red rash spreading around my eyes. My skin, used to $5 coconut oil as moisturizer, was angrily rebelling against the $100 cream Lona had just carefully applied.

"Oh, that's no problem!" she replied, fiddling around with more containers. "When that happens, you just put on this cream to fix it."

A cream designed to fix the problem that only existed because . . . oh, never mind.

"See—much better now!"

Lona devoted herself to the remainder of my facial without a hint of a sales pitch, as we chatted about her Hawaiian home. She then wrapped the tiny brushes in a tissue and, after a furtive glance over her shoulder, tucked them into my bag.

"Thank you, Lona," I said, acknowledging her expression of gratitude.

"Oh, thank *you*!" she beamed. "Enjoy the rest of your time in the United States!"

When there are players heavily invested in the further diminution of self-esteem, whether for money (e.g., the fashion and beauty industries casting normal aspects of a woman's appearance as problems, which you then need to pay to fix) or sex (e.g., a whole segment of the pick-up industry based on targeting women with low self-esteem and subtly insulting them, all to get them into bed), it becomes difficult to remain immune. This is especially the case should you have started from a position where you have experienced emotional trauma, or repeated knocks to your sense of self.

This, by the way, has very little to do with what you "attract." You do not need to internalize any blame if others try to undo you for *their* own gain.

However, this is not the end of the story. The first level of agency is the universal ability to choose to respond to your situation or circumstances. The classic articulation of this ability comes from *Man's Search for Meaning* author Viktor Frankl, who powerfully wrote, "Between stimulus and response, there is a space. In that space is our power to choose our response. In our response lies our growth and our freedom"—choosing a response being all the more compelling because Frankl wrote of his experiences in a Jewish concentration camp in the 1930s.[46] Frankl illustrates that you *can* still choose how to respond to a situation, even if it is ghastly beyond human comprehension, and is certainly not of your making in the first place. Second-order agency assumes that you have the resources, both inner and external, to make constructive changes in your life. You do not need to be a millionaire to make said changes, and I write with an expectation that you do have some degree of second-order agency if you are reading this book.

In order to respond effectively, we must trust that there is a better way. We must trust ourselves: that we know what is and is not good for us. We must trust that our bodies are beautiful, our selves sovereign, and that our souls do not exist as pawns in other people's games. When we engage with discernment and self-reflection, we must trust that our interpretations and feelings are valid and real, even if challenged by others.

Trust is the focal practice for the Gibbous Moon phase. It is not uncommon to find this the most challenging phase of the Moon cycle—the Moon moves toward its peak, but has not actually reached it yet. So often in life we rush to climax, partly because we do not feel comfortable in the in-between phases of life, and partly because we are so prone to constant doing that suspended motion is unfamiliar. Just being, trusting that we are okay, and understanding that being is an essential part of the cycle, demand our presence, rather than the increasing distractions of our modern existence.

Pausing at this Moon phase is where the "ick" can emerge. It is where we learn how to sit with the darkness, the shadow—to listen, deeply, to the cry and the hum within our heart, the rumble inside our womb, the ache in our back, the expansion in our lips. And then the deeper knowing, working its way up from our belly, from our dreams, knowledge from our deep subconscious blazing into our conscious mind—as anyone who has a meditation or contemplation practice will attest, this can only come when you are not trying to force it.

You do not become comfortable with discomfort—this is an oxymoron. Being with discomfort is not a destination or goal that you can check off the list; that is not the point. However, your *capacity* to be uncomfortable can expand, and, with it, your resilience and openness. From this ability to *be* with what is in our bodies grows the seed of trust. That trust is a trust of the ebb and flow of the universe, a trust of our sisters, and ultimately, a much deeper trust of ourselves. The Yin phases are the constant reminders for us to practice *being*—and it does take practice.

WHAT DOES A YIN PHASE LOOK LIKE?

A Yin phase does not mean stopping altogether. These phases involve an invitation to consider how we approach our work. Yin phases can be sweet, regular reminders to consider whether or not we are applying old patterns of intense achievement to our daily lives, and to consider modifying our approach if we find ourselves doing this.

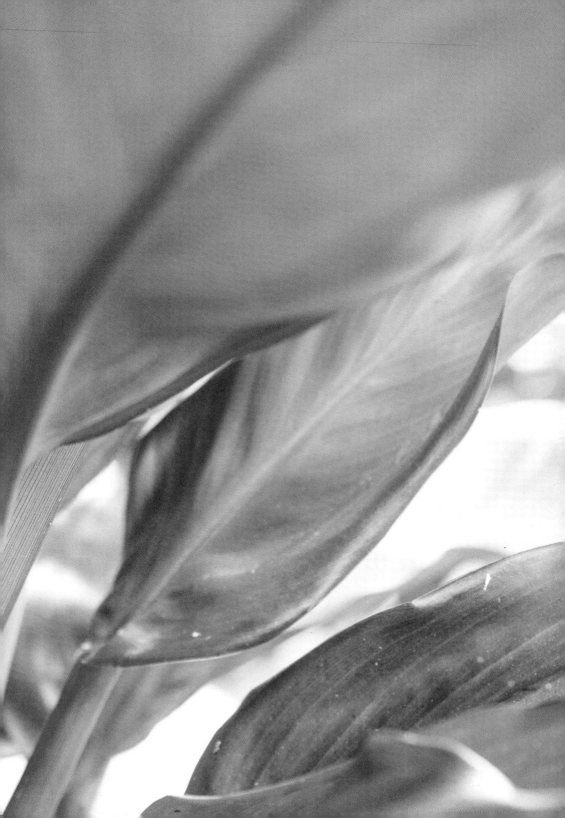

Remember that Yin and Yang phases are always relative, rather than absolute, terms. What this means is that these Yin phases will always be relative to what is going on in your life, as well as to your New Moon. Your Yin phase might look different from someone else's Yin phase. Your Yin phase will *definitely* look different from your Yang phase.

Asking what do we *do* during a Yin phase is very natural for us because we are such *doing* creatures, and we are living in a culture and a society where there is a lot of doing going on all the time. We are so conditioned around the doing that it can be difficult for us to even phrase the question in another way.

What we are really asking is:

How can we BE in a yin phase?

The Yin phases are not fantasy states, divorced from reality. These do not involve just sitting in bed and drinking cups of tea all day, or chilling out with piña coladas on a tropical beach. We all have responsibilities; we have bosses or clients; many of us have children or others dependent on us.

A Yin phase can be the time to notice your temptation to lean forward and to push to get things done. Examples of this include thinking, "Oh, I'll just keep on going and get the laundry finished" or "Just one more e-mail before I shut the laptop" or "Before I go home from work, I'll just get this one thing done." There is, and always will be, a never-ending mountain of things to do in work and life—a Yin phase invites you to witness your approach, to look at your process, and to see what it feels like to *not* push yourself for once (and to not beat yourself up about not pushing).

You can always move forward at the next Yang phase: the essence of a Yin phase is to practice being kind to yourself, and witness where you are not already. In this practice, we start to unwind our shadow patterns around achievement and what is motivating us.

During this Yin phase, you might observe where you do tend to just try to get things done—just try to push forward, just try to do that little bit too much—and then pay for it later because you end up burning out and exhausting yourself, or you do not execute it as well as you otherwise would have with refreshment and rest.

Studies have demonstrated that overwork and perfectionism lead to everything from diminishing performance to not being able to read facial expressions, to burnout, to being lost in the weeds of a project and unable to see the bigger picture.[47] There are times in life where we will have greater burdens and experience sleep deprivation; it is not always our choice. But the next time you consider "just pushing through," ask yourself whether you *do* have a choice to pull back even a little. Consider the long game: if you're sick, you will be less effective at work in the short term, and you will probably also be less effective in the longer term because your illness will limp along for additional days. If you keep pushing through when you are absolutely exhausted, you may reach the point of collapse—at which point you are taken out of action altogether, which is not helpful for you or anyone reliant on you.

Again, resting and restoring are not "nice to haves"; they are essential. What does this look like?

Start working with Yin phases in a low-risk environment.

Examples of exercises for a Yin phase:

❭ **Go for a slow walk** rather than a run, spin, or high-intensity workout.

❭ **Plan to stay home** and meditate (or read or take a bath), rather than going to the pub.

❭ **Find a role model** who is very Yin. Notice how she operates.

If you are in business:

❭ **Try scheduling most appointments** for Yang phases.

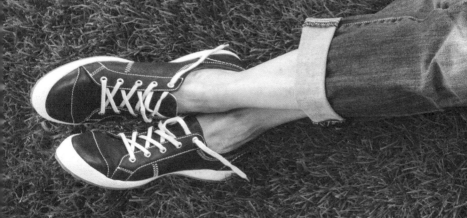

Resting
and *restoring*
are not
"nice to haves";
they are
essential.

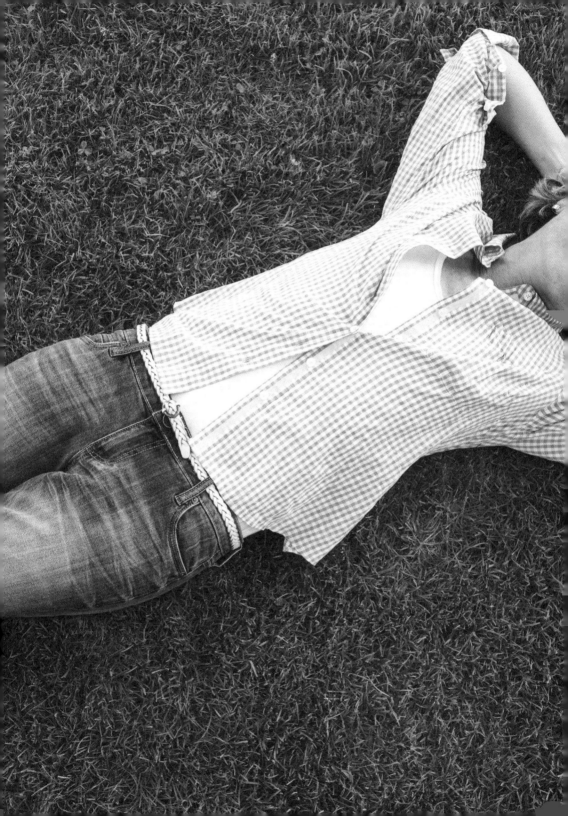

If you are at work:

> ❭ **Consider what you could hold over** until the next day.

For your kids:

> ❭ **Mindfulness practice**—consciously turn your awareness to three things that you can see, then three things that you can feel, smell, taste, and touch.

> ❭ **Set out a few art prompts** in the evenings for the kids to do in the mornings. Nothing overengineered, just, for example, a few feathers, a toilet-paper roll, and some tape, so your kids can start the day smiling.

In your day-to-day life:

> ❭ **Sit with your intention.**

> ❭ **Journal.**

> ❭ **Breathe deeply** into your belly.

> ❭ **Massages** (yes, there are good reasons to take massages as these lower cortisol, and raise dopamine and serotonin).

> ❭ **Practice self-care, however that looks for you**—baths, an early night, rest, etc.

What not to do in a Yin phase:

> ❭ **Push yourself,** if that is your proclivity.

> ❭ **Tell yourself,** "I'll just keep going till I get through this."

> ❭ **Feel guilty** for looking after yourself.

TRUST

The focal point for this phase is trust. Trust is not the same as blind faith, and trust definitely does not involve being reckless. For example, if you were not an experienced tightrope walker, you would not leap onto a wire strung between two high-rise buildings and "trust" that you will be held upright by unseen forces. Trust is not quitting your job without a plan and expecting a million dollars to rain down from the sky. These things involve you both abdicating your personal responsibility and ignoring Earth rules.

To the contrary, trust means taking deep responsibility, and in order to do that, you need to know yourself. You need to understand your terrain. You need to be able to situate yourself within that terrain.

This phase does not always make sense to our rational minds, and it does not work if we approach the phase with a defined objective—for example, if we feel sadness and strive to make our sadness go away. The paradox is that our sadness will mostly likely pass once we feel it, but as a by-product. Trusting involves feeling it all—knowing that it is *okay* to feel it all—just to feel it, and to trust what you feel.

When you start to trust yourself, you will be challenged to the ends of the Earth. Life's funny like that. If you say that you do not need external validation, you might just find that you are repeatedly invalidated before you settle into that state of being. If you practice the exercises in this chapter, you will not only become more open, grounded, and durable; you will become a force to be reckoned with.

ALEX

Alex is a mother of two gorgeous girls, living in a cute house built with her artistic husband in Canberra, Australia—her hometown. She studied English literature and then education in college. She was a fabulous primary school teacher before she burned out and moved into government to work on public education policy. A keen reader and a wonderful French cook, Alex has many passions, including music. Once the lead singer for an indie band, she now runs a community choir in her hometown (with an exquisite voice and keen ear for lyrics, she is a charismatic performer and plays a mean glockenspiel).

Alex's urge to take care of others has led her to study life coaching, and she is hoping to set up a business that allows her to both work more flexible hours and give more hands-on care to her small children. However, the juggling act does tend to exhaust her: family, work, study, a potential future business, spiritual questing, and the extracurricular—where does it end? Juggling full-time work with study, family, and community obligations means that Alex is constantly tired. She gets colds and flus with regularity, and berates herself when she becomes snippy with those she loves.

Alex's recent New Moon intentions attend to this. Her intention for the current month is, "I feel my body deeply *relax* as I courageously fill my *own* cup." After many months of following the Lunar Abundance practice—setting her intention, and noticing this intention take off well—Alex sees a pattern emerge. At the Gibbous Moon phase each month, she feels lost, overwhelmed, and confused. Every time.

After a while, Alex realizes that the Yin phases show her how much she pushes herself relentlessly to be the perfect person, the perfect mother, the perfect wife, the perfect employee, and the perfect community leader. Her cup is brimming over with actual responsibilities, to be sure; but, in addition to this, she spends a great deal of time trying to control her reality. She does not trust that things can function without her giving 100 percent, which wears on her adrenals. She does not feel that she will be taken seriously if she does not give everything she has. She does not trust that she can live in the gray. She does not trust that she will be supported to "do" life differently. She wants to give more than she is physically capable of giving, and to be the best at *everything*, which takes a lot of energy that she cannot afford to spend. This mentality traps her in a cycle of weariness-overwhelm-collapse-recover-weariness.

Sound familiar?

This brings us to more and less effective ways of experiencing Yin.

 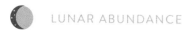

MORE AND LESS EFFECTIVE YIN

In the same way that we met the more and less effective ways that Yang played out in the previous chapter, in this chapter we meet the ways of being more and less effective Yin.

	LESS EFFECTIVE YIN	MORE EFFECTIVE YIN
Being	Controls	Allows uncertainty
Restoring	Helpless, overwhelmed	Nurture self and others
Listening	Too timid to speak	Hears and collaborates
Receiving	Reciprocates	Accepts with boundaries

Where might you be playing out less effective Yin in your life?

In this Moon phase, we explore the sense of being able to be with uncertainty—to be with the mystery. Brené Brown teaches that the ability to be with the unknown is a feature of effective leaders, or indeed, anyone living wholeheartedly. And here's the kicker: trust does not mean that nothing bad will happen. In *Rising Strong*, Brown writes, "If we are going to put ourselves out there and love with our whole hearts, we're going to experience heartbreak. If we're going to try new, innovative things, we're going to fail. If we're going to risk caring and engaging, we're going to experience disappointment."[48]

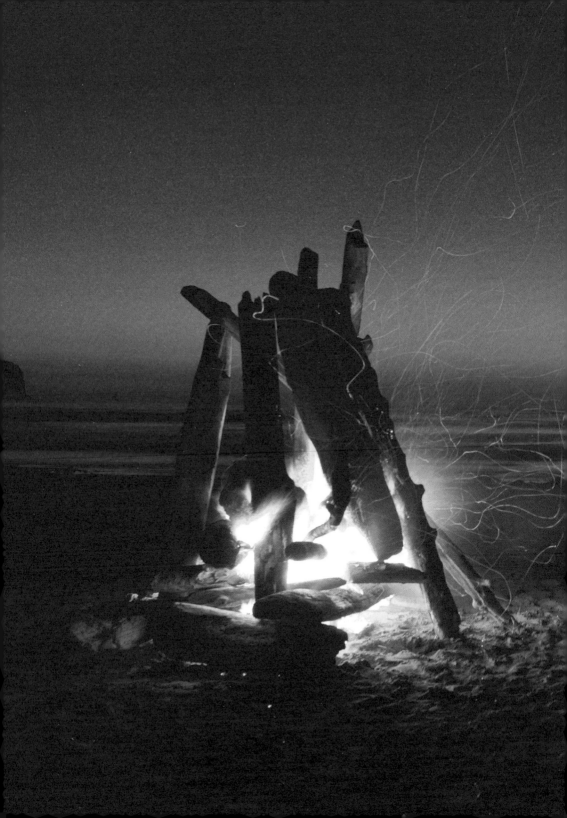

The ability to be
with the unknown
is a feature of
effective leaders,
or indeed, anyone living
wholeheartedly.

In other words, it is not a matter of *if* we will experience the "bad"; it is a matter of *when*. Trusting that you are supported and cared for, and that life is ultimately perfect, is not the same thing as never encountering sadness, anger, desolation, grief, loss, embarrassment, or fear. Trust means that you will open to life knowing that you will experience situations and emotions that bring you to your knees, and not shying away from these or modifying your reality to avoid them.

Learning to cultivate discernment means, however, that you will become better at ascertaining which situations should rightfully earn your trust. This means finding safe spaces and opening your heart—especially once you have built your strength, resilience, and support networks. It means carefully and mindfully finding the places, the relationships, and the situations where you are able to begin to play with these concepts.

Trust is essential to an abundance mind-set; trust is knowing that you are resourceful and supported, knowing that there are many who want to help, and owning your own part in the process by ripening, opening, and making good decisions.

Trust comes from going within to cultivate a sense of connection with ourselves.

I encourage you to start with something low-risk in order to find the situations where the sky will not fall, for example, if you're not pushing yourself—if you are being kind to yourself, if you are relaxing, if you are chilling out a little bit. It may even be that you are able to perform or deliver or create in a way that is actually far better.

When we start to trust that we are good enough and *that we are already enough,* a world starts to open up to us. No one else can give that world to us—we cannot pay for someone else to activate this for us through a weekend-long energy workshop or goddess training. It is not summoned forth by donning crystal pendants, as lovely as this may be. Trust comes from going within to cultivate a sense of connection with ourselves, so that we may build our own resilience and inner strength. It will feel murky and tender at first, and there will be discomfort as we start to feel into the uncertainty. However, uncertainty is not comfortable. The more that you accept this, the faster you will embrace reality and stand strong in your power; you will cultivate a sense of your own knowing, and develop discernment for right action when it is time to move.

Trust is also an expression of the Yin.

For example, when she's at the office, Alex likes to get things done to a certain standard by a certain time. What she finds when she pulls back and does *not* go above and beyond for a garden variety report, she meets the deadline, picks up her kids from child care on time, makes dinner, and finds the next morning that the report was well received. She did not need to go that extra mile on that particular report, which then opens up space for her to dedicate herself more fully to the next piece of work in the next (Full) Moon phase: a brief that goes up to the Minister for Education with her name on it.

Down with another cold the next week, Alex accepts her limits and asks for help with her community choir. The first person she asks says no—she is too busy herself. Alex feels despondent and guilty for reaching out, but tries again. The next person says, *Of course!* The third person she asks mentions that she has two girlfriends who have wanted to gain experience leading a community organization. They ask others. Before long, a committee of nine is running the choir, plus a musical team of five. The team loves being involved, and all are amazed that Alex used to do it all alone. Now she is grateful that she has created a beautiful community in Canberra, and is able to just arrive and sing on Thursday evenings, then go home for an early night.

This is trust in action: being intentional about what we want and then drawing back, being brave enough to ask for help when we need it, and, most important, being determined enough to persevere if at first we do not succeed.

We may expect that the universe shall instantly reward us for our realization, but usually we are then presented with a test. Once we pass the test, it is a whole new story. This is where we start to flow. It becomes more obvious to us when we may be overdoing things—where we may be controlling, or scripting, our reality. We start to realize what is preventing us from following the natural rhythms of life, knowing that we will be looked after and that everything is okay, even if it does not pan out quite how we thought it would.

CONCLUSION

When you start to consciously work with the Moon cycle, you may find that the Gibbous Moon Yin phase is one of the most challenging. This may be because it is the one that is most at odds with the way that we are used to living in the West. It *requires* us to put distractions to one side, to open to the mystery, and to feel. And then what we feel may not feel good at all—at least at first. We may make missteps and realize that we need to exert more effort in a certain area.

Of course, part of the process is to embrace all that is with an open heart. This is how we start to release subconscious stumbling blocks in a very gentle way, without problematizing the wrinkles around our eyes or in the fabric of our soul. This is how we start to *know* things; this is how we increasingly draw the right people, situations, and opportunities toward us to help make our intentions take form in the real world.

This emerges through the experience—not the fantasizing about it.

It's no coincidence that this Moon phase follows that of discernment. Cultivating discernment, intuition, and finding right action throughout is one of the aims of this lunar practice. Happily, the Moon cycle repeats, so these are concepts that you will continue to work with over time as you go deeper and deeper into the practice and deeper into the mystery, where you will find unexpected treasure and delight within you.

Summary

> Trust is the focal practice for this phase—trust of the ebbs and flows of the universe, trust of our sisters, and ultimately, trust in ourselves.

> It is key to learn to pause at this Moon phase—to learn to sit with the darkness and the shadow.

> It is not about becoming comfortable with discomfort, but rather expanding your capacity to be uncomfortable, as well as expanding your resilience and openness.

> We also learn where we should not trust—trust is not the same as blind faith. Cultivating discernment will help us work out which situations are right for us to trust.

> This phase is about exploring the sense of being able to be with uncertainty and mystery, to learn to trust that you are supported and cared for, and that you are already enough.

> Trust comes from going within in order to cultivate this sense of connection to ourselves, and to build up our own resilience and inner strength.

> Embrace all that is with an open heart.

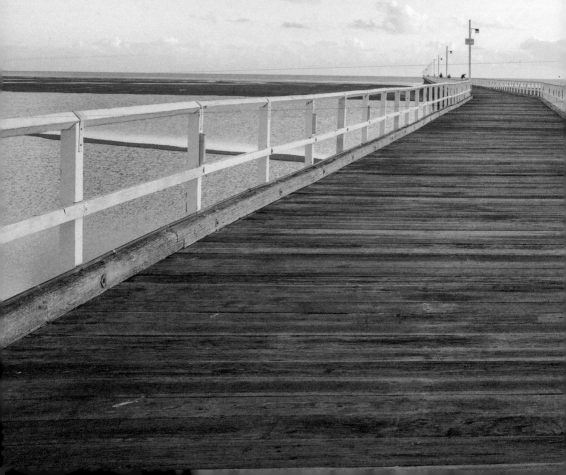

Trust

is not the same as

blind faith.

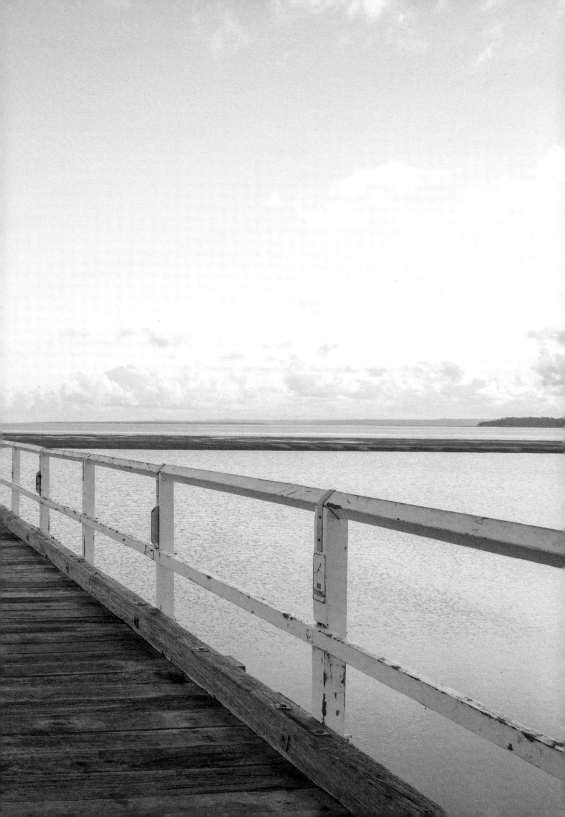

I am rooted but I flow.[49]

—VIRGINIA WOOLF

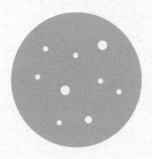

Full Moon

Have you ever been deep in nature at the time of the Full Moon?
The Full Moon is brilliant when seen from anywhere, but when I first *really* connected with this Moon phase in all its glory, I was out in nature, well away from any streetlights. I was flabbergasted—and I had been working closely with the Moon for many years by that point. There are layers and layers to this lunar practice, and this was one of the times that I went a lot deeper into the mysterious depths of lunar living and loving.

I had taken a camping trip out in the remote Australian bush with some friends one Easter. After dinner one evening—there had been violins and chai, dancing and entertaining conversation—it came time for this introvert to retreat back to her tent. As I moved away from the light of the bonfire to the camp, which was nestled among a grove of gumtrees, I noticed that the light from my flashlight was unnecessary. I looked around, and then up, and my jaw dropped. The Moon, just shy of full, had risen high in the sky and was lighting up my all my surroundings. The semi-arid landscape rolled out before my eyes in every direction, beautiful, even populated as it was by a smattering of kangaroos and a Portaloo.

Oh, I breathed. *Now I get it.*

Moonlight shone down upon my uplifted face as sudden shots of insights about my intentions unfurled in my awareness. The moment was visceral. The full sensation transcended words; my heart opened to hopes and dreams and mystery as I experienced the full majesty of the moment.

I realized, too, that I was experiencing that moment from a different angle—I had encountered a Paschal Full Moon while looking up at the sky, rather than down at a chart or at a calendar of dates (the Paschal Full Moon is the Full Moon associated with Easter). The lunar influence in the West is subtle, but remains present: it's there for us to notice and remember, if we pay attention.

That encounter also reminded me that our viewing lens shifts and expands when we become present to what is actually going on around us. We can expand our vision to 360 degrees. Sometimes I can get inspired by, but then a little enmeshed in, heady ideas and concepts—defaulting back to old patterns—but this moment served as a reminder that Moon wisdom comes best through pure perception: through *felt* experience.

The Full Moon is the culmination point of the Moon cycle. Every cycle waxes and wanes; every cycle has a beginning point, a surge, and a time when it winds back to darkness. This is the nature of all cyclical living.

The climactic point of the Moon cycle corresponds with the transition from youth to maturity in the life cycle, ovulation in the menstrual cycle, the peak of summer with the solstice, and the breathtaking glow of sunset in the day's cycle.[50] Demetra George writes that "the fruit embodies the full actualization of the essence of the seed"[51] planted at the New Moon—our intention, of course.

Everything is illuminated under the light of the Moon when it blooms to full. The creative life-force energy of the Moon cycle is at its maximum. If we have been nurturing our intention throughout the entire cycle, this climaxing lunar energy becomes our metaphorical pasture in which to grow and expand.

The Moon phases show us the Moon's shifting relationship to the Sun as it appears from Earth. The Full Moon is the point at which the Moon is directly opposite the Sun, on the other side of the Earth.

As the Sun's rays catch the Moon's surface at the cycle's zenith, the Moon fully reflects the light of the Sun back down to Earth.

The Full Moon also captivates our attention because the Moon is literally in full visual bloom; this is different than at other times in the Moon cycle. Recall that the Moon is physically opposite the Sun at the Full Moon; in this phase, the Moon rises at Sunset and sets at Sunrise. At other times throughout the Moon cycle, the Moon will rise throughout the day and night, depending on how close it is to the Sun as it orbits the Earth. During the early and late stages of the Moon cycle, the Moon appears from the perspective of Earth to be traveling more closely with the Sun, so you might catch sight of the Moon during the times that the Sun is visible, during the day or evening, rather than at midnight (the direction at which the Moon will rise depends on the season and hemisphere).

The system still works if you cannot see the Moon (whether at day or at night), say, because it is too cloudy or foggy. Recall that, in this practice, the Moon represents our feelings and subconscious worlds. While the image of the Moon can be a useful trigger for us to come within, the deeper work occurs in our internal feeling world. This is within *you*, and can be accessed wherever you are, whether or not the Moon is visible in the sky.

TIME TO HARVEST

Folklore from across the ages tells us that if you plant seeds by setting an intention at the New Moon—and, I would add, if you nourished those seeds throughout the waxing half of the Moon's cycle by following the steps set out at each of the Moon phases—then this Moon phase is the one to reap your harvest.

What may seem to magically materialize at this Moon phase will always be preceded by dedicated work. Much goes on beneath the visible surface.

You know that is the case for any kind of magic, right?

If you have come this far in the practice, you understand that it is not merely a matter of thinking about riches and treasure, and having these pour down upon you. As you well know, that is fantasy, a common trap that will keep you stuck.

In the Lunar Abundance practice, you are learning how to make things look "magical" on the surface. At the Full Moon phase, if you have been following this practice, you have shown up. You have collaborated with the situations, people, and opportunities around you over the past two weeks of the waxing Moon cycle—you have done so in real life, in real time. You are *co-creating*, continuing to take effective action to bring your intention into form and to shape your dream life.

ANOTHER YANG PHASE

As the Full Moon is another Yang phase, it is time to take action at this time—particularly if we have taken a breather in the preceding Gibbous Yin phase.

In our metaphorical system, the light that shines down on Earth is at the Full Moon phase and the path ahead is well defined.

If we are on track, that is.

The next steps for us to take now become obvious. It also may now be time to enjoy the fruits of our labors as things start to come into being.

But what if we have stumbled off the proverbial trail? If so, it may be time for us to course-correct.

The meaning behind this metaphor is most palpable when you get out from behind your screens, go outside at the Full Moon, and look up at night.

Deep in nature, connected to the Earth, away from city lights, distraction, and noise—this is when you will experience a greater appreciation of what is involved at this key phase of the lunar cycle. The path forward is literally *lit*. And you can feel it, with your senses ablaze: this is the time that you are able to fully experience and hold the emotional intensity that is flowing for you now.

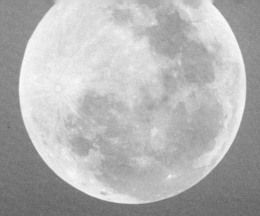

How might you *get outside* of the city at the next *Full Moon?*

Check the calendar to find dates for upcoming Full Moons.

Could you *plan a getaway?* Even a simple *camping trip?*

EMOTIONAL STABILITY

The Full Moon phase is most enjoyable *if* you have been paying attention to the ebbs and flows of the waxing Moon cycle and all the Moon phases up to this point.

It is also the Moon phase where people are most likely to start talking about how the Moon made them do it. Of course, the Moon does not *make* you do anything. You have agency over how you feel. You respond to it. You claim it.

One of the points of this practice is to work in harmony with nature to find your own natural rhythm and flow—not to bow down to external influence.

The more you pay attention to your feelings, the more sensitive you will become. But being sensitive does *not* mean that you need to lie on the floor and wail at the Full Moon. You can be sensitive, feel a great deal, and still function beautifully (for help with this, try one of the contained Full Moon release ceremonies outlined on page 158).

You will feel the Full Moon phase, more and more over many Moon cycles (a reminder that when I talk about feelings, I mean physical sensations in your body). You may feel an expansion in your chest, a rushing of energy through your veins, or a tingling in your legs. You may also feel an intensifying of emotions, or attribute new meaning to them: to anger, grief, fear, sadness, love, joy, elation, inspiration, delight, hope, gratitude, and deep peace. You may feel more energy, or you may feel less. There is no right or wrong to what you feel—our task here is to experience what is going on, get curious, feel, and if we then choose to, respond rather than *react*, for example, out of frustration or anxiety.

This phase is also about cultivating self-knowledge—you will see where old, subconscious patterns play out in real time.

We can get off the emotional roller coaster at the Full Moon by beginning our lunar practice at the start of the lunar cycle, two weeks earlier at the New Moon, and then paying close attention throughout the lunar cycle. This way, we ensure that we are riding the entire wave and experiencing the peak in context, not just dropping in at the crest and splashing around in a mad panic.

THE ACT OF LETTING GO

Letting go is as essential an abundance principle as the ushering in of the new. Why? Because being in the flow requires us to have the space to receive. One of the constants of life is change, after all.

Letting go at this phase could be anything from clearing out your cupboards, deleting old files from the computer hard drive, letting go of old systems in our businesses, and also clearing out old beliefs: we let go of old ways of relating to our finances or stories about what happened to us in childhood.

Terrible things do happen, of course. However, there comes a time and a place for you to realize when you are still holding on to what happened in a way that is preventing future expansion and the growth of your heart.

The act of letting go has numerous health and well-being benefits. Societies all around the world have customs of confession and disclosure.[52] It has been demonstrated that the use of writing or journaling to express and release emotions can greatly assist in the processing of stressful or traumatic life events.[53] Emotional release has a profound effect on our physicality: one study has shown that emotive response through swearing may actually lessen the experience of physical pain.[54] Conversely, it has been demonstrated that withholding our emotions poses a great health risk. One study found that a link existed between emotional suppression and cardiovascular and cancer mortality.[55] Moreover, it is not just the release of emotion that may provide health benefits. Letting go of possessions and a materialistic focus supports health. Studies demonstrate that individuals are more likely to experience happiness through experiential spending than the accumulation of material possessions[56] (though this effect may depend on an individual's starting point).

Once we have recovered, our experiences can be the fuel for resilience: to create lasting change, for ourselves and for others. As you focus on what you want to bring into your life, you may need to create space.

And how to do that? Keep reading and you'll find three easy ways.

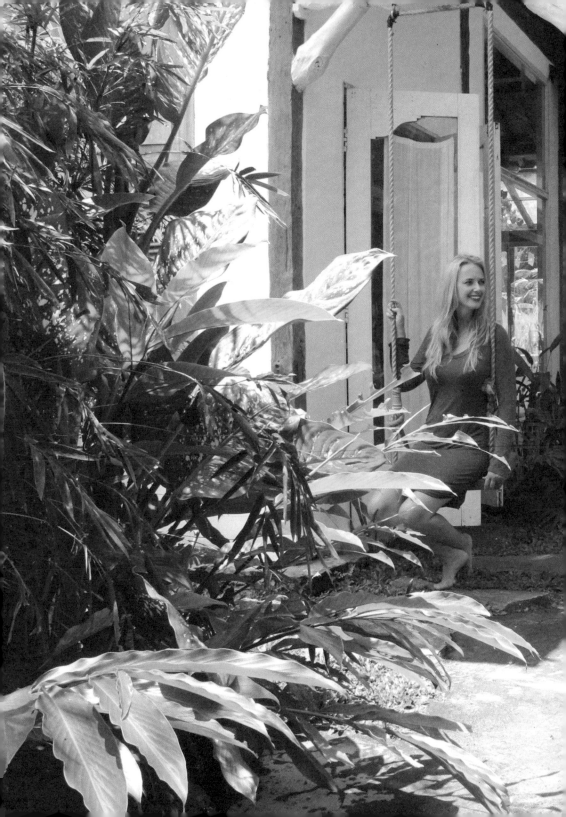

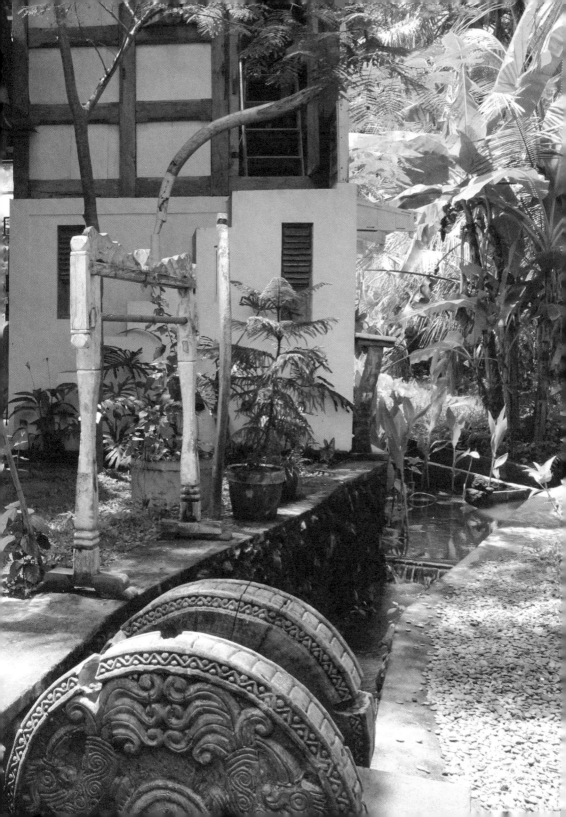

What might release look like in real life?

Katie's New Moon intention was to welcome in her tribe. She wanted to find a new group of soul sisters. Happily married with a kind and caring husband, she felt a growing sense of isolation in her own life, especially when following social media profiles of famous life coaches. Journaling at the Full Moon, she realized that deep down she did not believe that women could truly support each other. Her experience growing up was that women were insecure, always jockeying for their own position in a hierarchy. Being carefully honest with herself, Katie realizes that this perspective may be affecting her own behavior with women and realizes that it is time to let this go if she wants to grow and experience truly loving and supportive relationships with other women. She decides to do a release ceremony on her previous beliefs (and to forgive her mother for her part in creating these). She takes the first step of reaching out to some women from her Sunday morning yoga class. Would they like to join her for a Full Moon ceremony? She feels a leap in her chest when three women say, *Oh, yes!*

Tai's New Moon intention was to feel the sizzle of a new romance. In fact, this had been her intention for the past three lunar cycles. She felt *ready*! After having followed all the steps throughout the Moon phases, at this Full Moon she finally came face-to-face with the realization that she had been pushing out of her conscious awareness: she was still blaming herself for the breakdown of her relationship with her ex-husband. Tai realized that she needed to forgive not just him but *herself* for not being the right match. She had to let go of the angst around this. Her second realization? That Internet dating is now a totally appropriate way to meet quality men looking for love. It really was time at this Full Moon to go ahead and set up that profile that she had been resisting.

Brigette's New Moon intention was to find a professional purpose that fit her higher aims in life. She works as an accountant, but she felt the life slowly being squashed out of her in this job. She racked her brains about what it was that she was here on Earth to do. She considered signing up for life coach training but nothing felt quite right; the dates weren't quite lining up, either. She did, though, love to practice Pilates at the studio next door to her firm: what started as a weekly practice evolved into almost daily visits. On the day of the Full Moon, a teacher who has been paying close attention to her progress approaches Brigette after class. "We are putting together a teacher-training program," she says. "Would you be interested in coming as a free beta-tester for us and giving us feedback? You would be the first to receive our studio certification at the end." Brigette had no intention to be a Pilates teacher. She has no idea where this may lead but realizes that her heart is crying out. "*Yes*," she says.

Lamisah's New Moon intention for this lunar cycle was to receive greater prosperity. What she realized at the Full Moon phase was that she had subconscious patterns relating to money that caused her to hold back from charging market rate for her reiki sessions, even though they had received glowing praise from her clients. Sitting in meditation with her New Moon intention one morning, Lamisah realized that deep down she believed that people could not be wealthy and do good in the world. While she had been complaining out loud that she did not have enough money to pay her rent, on a deeper level she believed that to receive proper payment for her sessions would corrupt their healing potential. At the Full Moon phase, Lamisah realizes that it is time to let go of these beliefs, then raise her prices—so that she could keep offering sessions to her clients, and not have to shut up shop altogether, exhausted and needing to return to her corporate career.

Take some time to be by yourself.

If you do not know what to release at the Full Moon, don't worry about it. This may take some time to bubble up from your subconscious. Take some time to be by yourself at this phase. You may wish to return to the New Moon Ceremony Checklist in the New Moon chapter for inspiration to set up a ceremony conducive to this type of self-inquiry and self-exploration.

Bring out your journal and pose a question for yourself: *What do I need to release now?* You do not need to know the answer. You can wait to see what, if anything, emerges as an answer. You can write or draw. Your work is for you. You don't need an exact response yet.

And remember, at the Full Moon you can just get friends together, eat, dance, and enjoy yourself. You do not need to go digging for issues—you can just have fun!

HOW TO RELEASE? FULL MOON CEREMONY

I'm a lover of simplicity, so you will find that these examples cut right to the quick.

However, follow your inspiration. You might like to create more ritual around these ceremonies.

And gathering a group of friends to join in the fun? Priceless.

Remember, though, while this may be lots of fun, it is only the icing on the cake. My view is not to miss the deeper point of release.

BURN BABY BURN

Write down on a piece of paper what is no longer serving you:

⟩ What is holding you back from your New Moon intention?

⟩ What are you afraid of?

⟩ What are you *really* afraid of?

⟩ Who are you angry at?

⟩ Who has slighted you?

⟩ What frustrates you?

Full Moon Release List

Full Moon Release List
(continued)

Who do you need to forgive? (Don't leave yourself off the list.)

》 **Get your pen** and purge onto the page.

》 **Then grab your matches**, your candle, and burn that list. (If you are inside, perhaps use a bowl, and have some water at the ready!)

》 **Even better:** gather a group of your sisters around a campfire.

Thrust your lists into the blaze and let 'em *burn*. Check in: how does that feel? Lighter?

WASH IT AWAY

Allow yourself to fully feel what is coming up for you at this time.

Write it down, talk it out, allow your body to fully immerse in the emotion. Then wash it off. Take a shower, frolic in the ocean, luxuriate in the bath, dance outside in the rain.

And of course, the oldie and goodie: cry it out. Crying can be incredibly cathartic, transmuting grief and pain as you literally let it go. Some types of tears can have functional purposes: ongoing secretions maintain the health of our eyes and remove foreign objects and irritations. There is, though, a category of tears that arise in response to emotions—perhaps unique to humans[57] and with far higher levels of serotonin than other tears.[58] Dr. Judith Orloff writes that emotional tears are in a very real sense the body's way of "purging stress and unhappiness" and reducing stress hormones.[59]

See, there is a point to crying, after all!

SHAKE YOUR BOOTY

This one you can do at home in your living-room, or even better yet, outside.

Or get together with friends and go out.

Crank your most hopping tunes, shake your booty, shake out your body, and get your whirl on. Bonus points for a big belly laugh: another wonderful way to get something off your chest is to see the *ridiculousness* of a situation.

HOW WILL YOU DESIGN YOUR FULL MOON CEREMONY?

I believe strongly in paying attention to results so that you can determine the effectiveness of this practice for yourself (discernment, yeah?). So pay attention to what starts to shift and change in your external world as a result of these simple release rituals.

CONCLUSION

At the Full Moon phase we practice emotional stability. We learn that we can be highly sensitive and *also stable*. In fact, I believe this is a feminine superpower: to be able to feel all the feels and to be able to hold them at the same time. This is the way to take wise action informed by our intuition, rather than exist in a state of constant reaction.

Feel all the feels and be able to hold them at the same time . . .

The Full Moon phase is also the time in the lunar cycle when we may start to reap what we have sown, and to release that which is holding us back from further abundance. Recall your New Moon intention at the Full Moon phase, cast your eyes forward and around, check in on your path, and take effective action.

Be ready to course-correct at this phase if it becomes apparent that you have wandered off in a direction not in alignment with either your New Moon intention or your larger objectives and goals. And stay open, in case you are presented with an opportunity different from what you had previously planned but in alignment with your desires. The best way to check is to see if you feel a physical expansion in your body and a resounding *yes* in your belly. (And, yes, it may be helpful to confirm that gut feel with the powers of reason, but no, it may not always make sense. It is up to you to measure up the risks involved and decide whether you can tolerate them.)

You do not need to throw caution to the wind altogether. Never do or receive anything that does not feel right to you, as we shall learn in the next chapter.

Stay aware and poised as you embrace your superpowers and learn to ride each cresting Full Moon with increasing levels of mastery and grace.

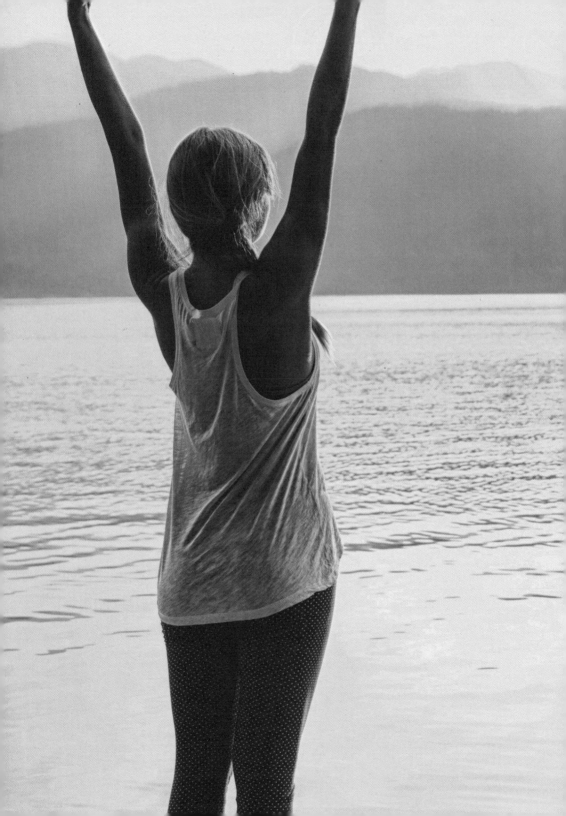

Stay *aware* and *poised*

as you embrace

your *superpowers.*

Summary

❯ The Full Moon is the culmination point of the Moon cycle. Remember, what may seemingly magically materialize at the Full Moon will always be preceded by dedicated work.

❯ The next steps to take may now be obvious. On the other hand, it may be time to enjoy the fruits of our work. If we are moving in a direction that is not conducive to our higher purpose, however, this may be the time to course-correct.

❯ Consider undertaking a Full Moon Ceremony to assist with the process of releasing—this could involve burning, washing away, or shaking it up!

❯ We can be stable *and* highly sensitive. This is the time to practice.

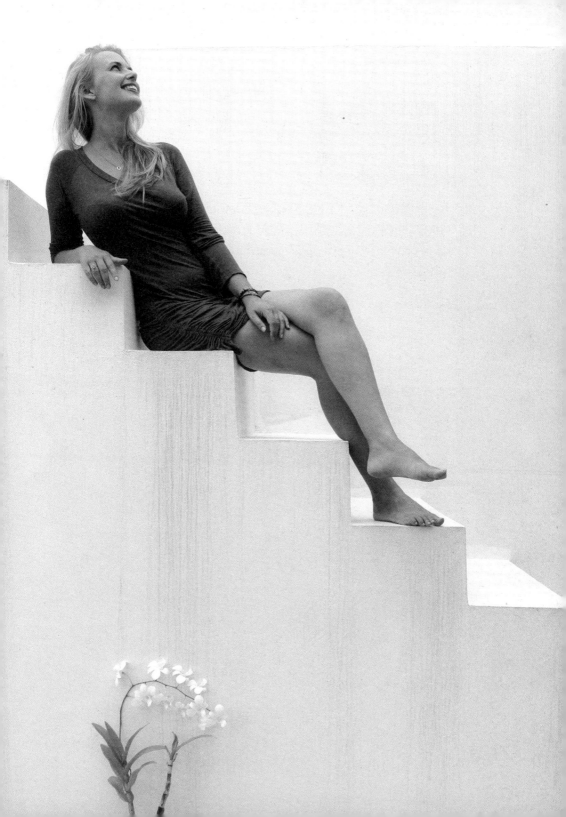

If you don't like something, change it.
If you can't change it, change your attitude.[60]

—DR. MAYA ANGELOU

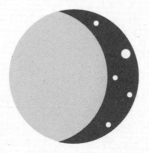

Disseminating Moon

At this phase, the Disseminating Moon phase—or the Waning Gibbous phase, as it is sometimes called—the Moon enters another Yin time, as she starts to make her way back from Full to New, from full illumination to deep darkness.

In the plant cycle, this is a time of fruiting; we reach maturity in our life cycle; the twilight emerges; and autumn or fall proceeds as we move beyond the period marked by the summer solstice.[61]

And what does that mean in relationship to our intention-setting?

One of the benefits of a Lunar Abundance practice is that it keeps you anchored and centered *all* the time. It is not just about setting your intention at the New Moon, celebrating at the Full Moon, and then neglecting your lunar love until it becomes trendy again.

The Moon is always there; she is always guiding us home to ourselves.

She *always* has something to offer.

Our job is to keep showing up and receiving this: consistently. What may seem insignificant on a daily basis in terms of attention and effort can have significant—and cumulative—effects over time.

The waning part of the cycle is not about checking out. Any practice requires devotion to yield results. So even after the excitement of the Full Moon, stay committed to your intention for the remaining three Moon phases of the cycle. Every single phase of the Moon cycle has an important part to play in this practice.

Any practice requires devotion to yield results.

Keep feeling it.

The emphasis of this lunar phase? To help us receive the fruits of our labor.

RECEIVING

Healthy receiving is a marker of high self-esteem. Being able to receive is key to creating greater abundance. And receiving graciously can bring enormous joy to another person. Both giving (Yang) and receiving (Yin) are essential to living and working effectively. However, those with low self-esteem may have difficulty receiving at all. They may also open the floodgates to receiving everything, without a filter, which can be dangerous.

As this Disseminating Moon phase is a Yin phase, we are focusing on receiving. We need to expand our receptivity container to be able to cultivate all types of abundance. We want this to be healthy, effective receiving that will enhance our well-being, whether it be financial, spiritual, romantic, or otherwise.

How? The first principle here is that it is important to receive *selectively*.

This is practical. If you devote yourself to an abundance practice (actually doing it, rather than just thinking about it), at some point you will find that you are flooded with opportunity. You will literally not be able to accept every invitation or even note or gift. You will not have capacity or time to do so.

You also may not *want* to receive some of the attention that you start to receive. If you open yourself up to romantic abundance, say, just because someone *wants* to compliment you does not mean that you need to receive that particular compliment from that particular person—however it was intended.

The point of this phase is also not to suggest that you should be open to receiving anything in any circumstance. Even things that initially seem appealing might require more consideration. Being aware of your boundaries and walking away are more than appropriate in these cases. You could also draw on support, if necessary.

At this Moon phase, we see the discernment principle operating again but in a different context. This is discernment in receiving, rather than in acting. This phase is not about opening the floodgates for receiving; that is an expression of *less effective Yin*. Be selective in how you receive by working out what you want to receive—first in advance (that is, by getting clear and setting an intention at the New Moon) and repeat that intention by reflecting as you go.

By all means, if your intention has flourished and is bearing fruit, then receive this and celebrate at the Disseminating Moon phase. If it does not yet seem to be in full flight, it may be that you are missing the small signs.

If you struggle with this phase, it is best to practice this principle in low-risk environments. Something as innocuous as accepting a compliment may be notoriously difficult for women—and deeply healing to practice—for the reasons described by Dr. Clarissa Pinkola Estés:

> *Although it could be a matter of modesty, or could be attributed to shyness—although too many serious wounds are carelessly written off as "nothing but shyness"—more often a compliment is stuttered around about because it sets up an automatic and unpleasant dialogue in the woman's mind. If you say how lovely she is, or how beautiful her art is, or compliment anything else her soul took part in, inspired, or suffused, something in her mind says she is undeserving and you, the complimentor, are an idiot for thinking such a thing to begin with. Rather than under-stand that the beauty of her soul shines through when she is being herself, the woman changes the subject and effectively snatches nourishment away from the soul-self, which thrives on being acknowledged.[62]*

Let's look at another low-risk example of practicing receiving.

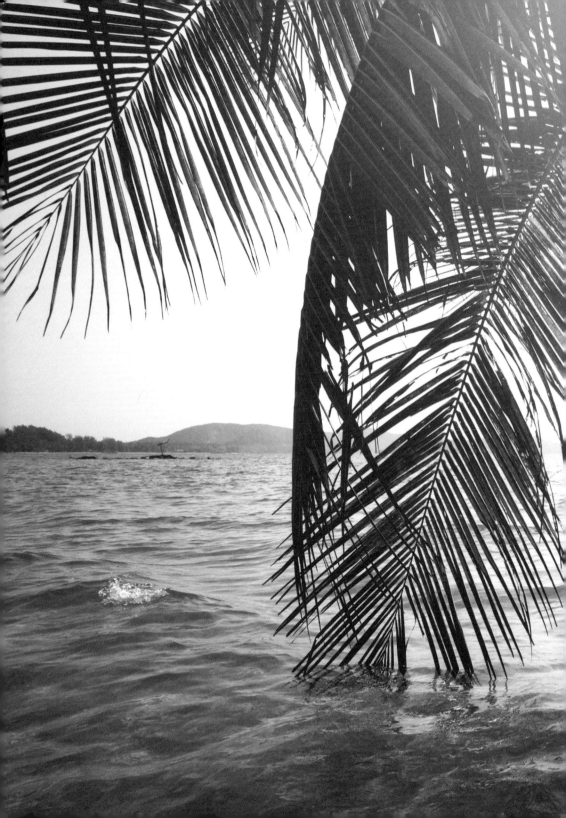

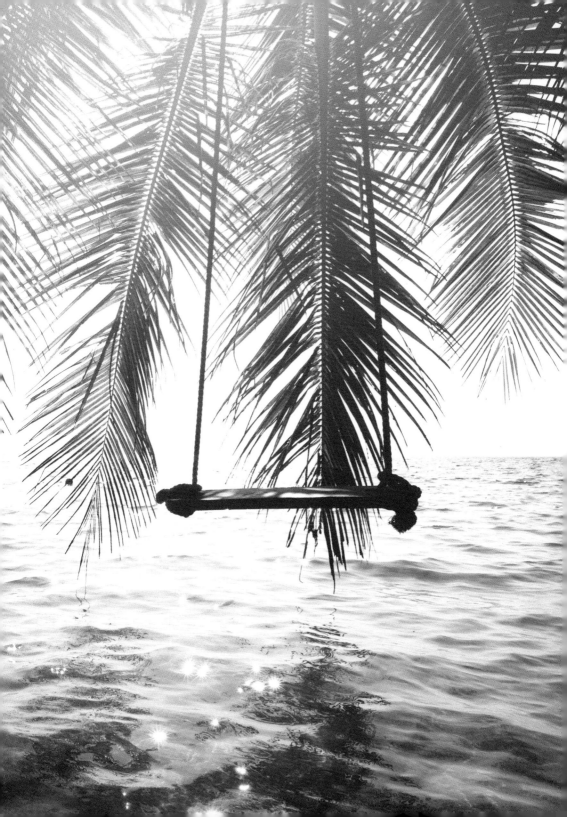

THE COFFEE

Jennifer set an intention at the New Moon in this lunar cycle on the theme of wanting to receive more support from men in her life. When she set her intention, she was secretly hoping that a certain man at her evening accounting class would give her a bit more attention, maybe even ask her out to dinner—but, hey, anything would be better than her current man drought!

At the Disseminating Moon phase, Jennifer's colleague Martin offers to buy her a coffee. Martin is not especially charismatic; in fact, since he started at the company a few months back Jennifer hasn't really had a chance to chat with him. It's obvious in this context that he's showing up to help with her intention, right? But given the busy swirl of Jennifer's life—plus the fact that Martin isn't immediately attractive to her—it might take a moment for the penny to drop.

Let's imagine Jennifer's automatic response to Martin, who's just asked if he can buy her a coffee:

Jennifer: No, no, I'll get it! I don't want you to have to go out in the cold!

Martin: No, really, it's fine. I'm going out myself.

Jennifer: Well, okay, but I feel bad. Here! Let me pay you back! (She scrambles in her purse.)

Martin: It's fine. It's just a couple bucks.

Jennifer: Oh but I have it! Wait! I almost have it!

Martin: (quietly rebuffed) Um, okay. Thanks. Almond milk, right?

Jennifer: (happy she didn't put Martin out) Yep!

AN ALTERNATIVE:

Martin offers to buy Jennifer a coffee.

Jennifer: Oh—really?

Martin: Yes, I'd love to!

Jennifer: Well, thank you, that would be wonderful. I didn't get much sleep last night and I have a mountain of paperwork to get through by lunchtime!

 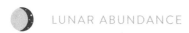

Martin: Awesome. Almond milk, right?

Jennifer: You remember!

Jennifer receives the coffee with a grateful smile.

ANOTHER ALTERNATIVE:

Martin offers to buy Jennifer a coffee.

Jennifer has just had her morning coffee. She could take or leave another one.

She recalls her New Moon intention about receiving greater support, though.

And she has just noticed on her Lunar Abundance planner that it is the Disseminating Moon phase.

And Martin—actually, she had never really looked closely at Martin before, but he has quite a nice smile.

Jennifer decides that this is a pretty low-risk scenario in which to practice receiving.

Jennifer: That would be really nice, Martin, thanks.

Martin: Awesome! Almond milk latte, coming right up.

ANOTHER EXAMPLE:

Martin offers her a coffee, but Jennifer does not feel like coffee.

Jennifer: Oh, that's a kind offer! I don't drink coffee in the afternoons, alas. It keeps me awake. I'll take you up on that next time, though!

Martin: Well, I'm headed to the coffee shop on the corner. I heard they do a mean hot chocolate. Can I get you one of those?

Jennifer: Well, sure. That would be nice! [Or, I'd love an orange juice, etc.].

EXAMPLE OF WHEN NOT TO RECEIVE THE OFFER

Jennifer's other colleague Jay has a habit of making up excuses to come over to her desk to chat, manufacturing things he can offer her and expecting her time in return. Jennifer tends to feel a guilt-charged urge to instantly respond when someone does something nice for her. Jay did buy her a coffee last week and then stood at the end of Jennifer's desk complaining about his car, work, and cousins. It wasn't until Jennifer finished drinking her coffee that she felt she could finally clear her throat and mention that she really *did* need to get back to work now.

Jay: Hey, Jennifer, I'm going to the coffee shop now. Want a coffee? [Jennifer decides the situation feels off-key.]
Jennifer: No, but thanks, Jay. I feel like getting some air. I'll get my own coffee soon.

Jay hovers for a beat, then walks off.

You can play this out in a variety of different circumstances, depending on your personal New Moon intention and life circumstances. These situations don't need to be about men wanting to give you something. You're wearing a new jacket? When your sister genuinely compliments you on it, can you take a moment to *receive* the compliment, to feel it in your chest, rather than say that you only bought it because it was on sale? When your client thanks you profusely for the change you helped effect in her life, can you give yourself (and *her*) the gift of allowing yourself to receive her gratitude? Don't rush to say that your advice was obvious and that anyone could have seen what needed to be done in her situation.

Be sure to take note of the small things. You might try journaling at the end of the day, for example, about what came into your life that day and what you're grateful for. *How will you be able to receive the big things when you are unable to receive the small joys of life?*

What's your receiving pattern?

 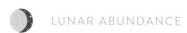

Is *yes* your first response

to *invitations, offers,* or *requests*

(and do you then notice that you *regret it later,*

or wonder why you are

not reaching your stated aims or objectives)?

Or

Is *no* your first response (and do you

then bemoan the *lack of abundance,*

soul sisters, healthy food,

or *romance* in your town)?

There is plenty of time for giving (and we focus on it in the next chapter), but in this Moon phase we are practicing being in the flow of receiving. When good things come into your life do you feel compelled to play them down—or to reciprocate? Or can you receive them just fine?

RECEIVING WITH GRATITUDE

Gratitude has been linked to changes in the brain activated by the "feel good" neurotransmitters, like serotonin and dopamine. More than helping us feel personally happy, though, studies have shown that gratitude helps us to strengthen and forge new social relationships. Those who regularly practice gratitude have been shown to be more helpful and altruistic toward others, so there are plenty of good reasons to embed more gratitude into your life.[63]

The most powerful receiving is that which is accompanied with the feeling of gratitude. We all can feel the difference between giving genuine thanks to someone—and for them to be insincere in their reply (perhaps because they themselves find it difficult to receive)—and giving our gift to someone whose ability to receive what we have to offer is deep, genuine, and heartfelt.

Heartfelt means exactly that: *feeling something with your heart.*

This is not a turn of phrase. It is a literal description. After all, feelings as understood in the Lunar Abundance practice are physical sensations in the body. When you feel gratitude, you may feel a warmth and expansion in your chest; you may feel movement of energy through your arms and legs. You may feel your hands and palms tingle. You may feel sensations elsewhere in your body. You may not feel any of this at all, at first—the invitation is to continue to feel, as you build up this sense over time, as you cultivate a closer integration between your mind and your body.

❭ **You can feel grateful for what you are receiving.** What is coming into your life right now?

❭ **You can also feel grateful for what you are yet to receive.** What have you not yet received but are hoping to receive? How does it feel to feel grateful for this?

❭ **You can feel grateful for the success of others.** Is your friend successful at something that you have been wanting to cultivate? How does it feel to feel grateful for her success?

Heartfelt means
exactly that:
*feeling something
with your heart.*

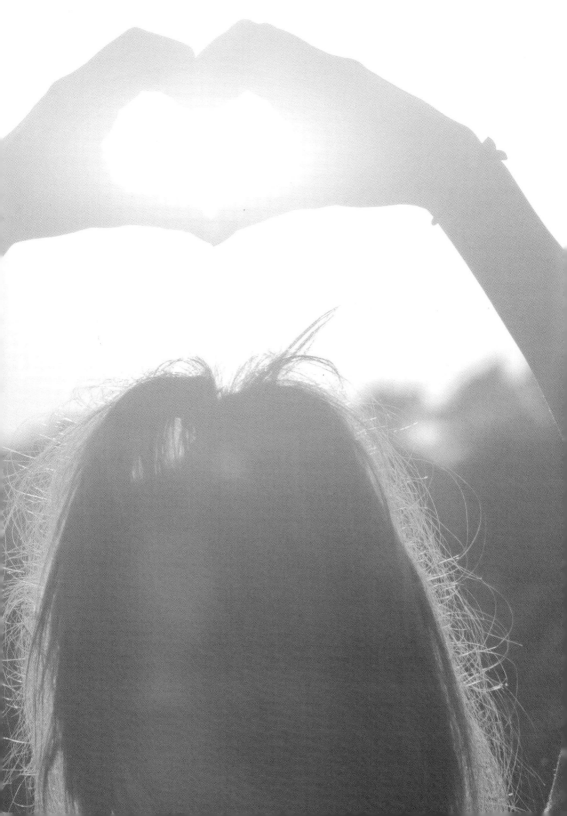

HOW TO NOT MISUSE GRATITUDE

Has someone ever suggested to you, in your hospital bed or after you pour out your emotional woes, that you should feel grateful for a challenge that will help you grow? That you should feel grateful for the death of your loved one, for a death fulfills a soul contract? That you should feel grateful that X did not happen (when Y did, and it was pretty horrible?).

This kind of response is incredibly annoying and may even be damaging. If you are someone who is susceptible to taking on responsibility, you may interpret it as an obligation to feel grateful for something awful in your life. As discussed below, a redemption narrative can be helpful in responding to the inevitable vicissitudes of life. But here is the thing: You do *not* need to feel grateful for terrible things—for example, a relationship with an abusive partner. We do not need to deploy gratitude in this type of dysfunctional situation. If someone is hurting you, don't work with gratitude as a way to settle for less than you are worth (which is, at a minimum, safety—nor should you have your self-esteem and well-being eviscerated). Reach out for support to help you leave the situation, whether through friends, family, colleagues, or crisis hotlines.

If you have suffered a loss, grief, or heartbreak, allow yourself to feel your pain, rather than numbing it or suppressing it. The invitation is not to "use" gratitude as a way to shortcut the messiness of this life. Life *is* messy. This can be one form of spiritual bypassing, a way of skipping the human experience by using spiritual or personal development concepts. Feeling our unresolved wounds fully can help us to deal effectively with our grief, trauma, or loss. These are topics covered by authors such as Chogyam Trungpa Rinpoche, John Welwood, Dr. Robert Augustus Masters, and by Dr. Azita Nahai in her *Trauma to Dharma* work (these and others are listed in the Resources section at the back of this book).

When you have felt your pain, experienced catharsis, and accepted it, and when you are out of crisis—when you are ready to move on, when you are truly ready—then feel grateful for what you learned, grateful for your ability to respond to pain and for those surrounding you who helped you through it.

The Hero's Journey—the monomyth described by Joseph Campbell—is a

 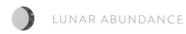

compelling story. It sells numerous books, movies, and rags-to-riches stories, but it has also been critiqued for a number of reasons, including that it does not fully encapsulate a woman's experience. Maureen Murdock outlines an alternative journey—cyclical, as opposed to the linear progression of the Hero's Journey—that modern women tend to undertake. Beginning in girlhood, a woman identifies with her father and rejects the feminine. She foregrounds masculine qualities to become successful in the external world until she meets her rejected feminine nature and descends to the dark goddess in a process of remembering and reclaiming the feminine. She then reintegrates her feminine self, eventually finding union between feminine and masculine in internal and external ways that honor both.[64] This ultimate integration and wholeness is found in other Jungian individuation work like that of Marion Woodman.[65] Related Heroines' Journeys are addressed in Barbara Stanny's *Sacred Success* and in the work of a number of other female authors.

Consider your own life through this lens. Does it ring True for you?

You do not always need a redemption narrative, or a narrative to your life at all. Another perspective involves recognizing that growth is inevitable and that it is possible for you to advance without struggling or overcoming adversity in every facet of your life. In fact, shaping your own past, present, and future into a "journey" or "story" is a peculiarly Western trait. However, elements of a redemption narrative *can* play a useful role in keeping your morale high—they can help you find meaning and purpose in the face of an otherwise incomprehensible world. Dan McAdams found in his research that successful entrepreneurs' "failures become part of the grand narrative of progress." In other words, those who had suffered difficulty tended to think "[t]hat had to happen, and I needed that setback, or I wouldn't have made this discovery."[66] Whether or not this is objectively true—and it may well be—this approach seems to fill a life with purpose and enjoyment.

Whether you choose to work with gratitude in this way, know that it is available to you. A mind-set of gratitude alone will not make your woes vanish in an instant. But feeling grateful will help you see the next step that you can take, and it will infuse you with optimism and confidence that you can take that step.

CONCLUSION

Receiving is a key Yin principle. The more you are able to receive in healthy and effective ways, the more you will be able to enter the flow of life, make others happy, cultivate abundance, and enjoy yourself a little more! There are principles regarding healthy and effective receiving that are worth following to avoid the less effective ways of being in Yin—to be so closed that you are unable to receive at all (not conducive to abundance!) or to be so open that you receive everything without discernment, preventing you from living in a purposeful and intentional way, able to focus on the aspects of life truly important to you.

And now that we have started to receive? It is time to give back.

Summary

❭ After the excitement of the Full Moon, stay committed to your practice for the remainder of the Moon cycle. The waning part of the cycle (and Yin phases in general) is not about checking out. Any practice requires ongoing devotion to yield results.

❭ The emphasis of this Yin phase is to help us receive. Receive selectively— as opportunity floods in, you will not be able to accept every invitation or you may not want to. Look to the return of the discernment principle: discernment in receiving and being, as well as giving or acting.

❭ Receiving is most powerful when accompanied by a feeling of gratitude.

❭ Elements of a redemption narrative, when working with gratitude, can be helpful in keeping up your morale and helping you to see the next step to take. There is no obligation to feel grateful for awful things going on in your life, however. Before reaching for gratitude, reach for support.

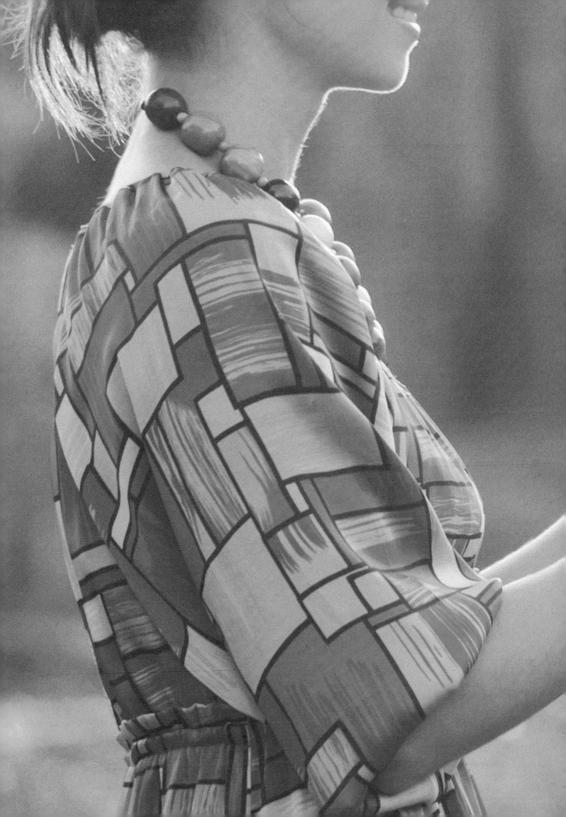

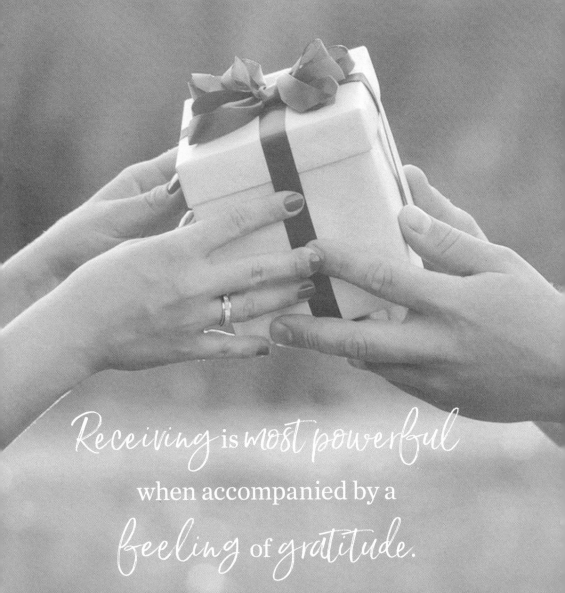

Receiving is most powerful
when accompanied by a
feeling of gratitude.

Until we can receive with an open heart, we're never really giving with an open heart. When we attach judgment to receiving help, we knowingly or unknowingly attach judgment to giving help.[67]

—DR. BRENÉ BROWN

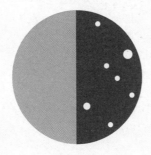

Third Quarter Moon

The Moon wanes even further now in the sky, back down toward the darkness of the New Moon as we enter the final Yang phase: the Third Quarter phase.

Our cycles are unique, but we have a habit of cycling *together*. Women living together certainly tend to synchronize.[68] But what of those who do not bleed? Only some women have a menstrual cycle, after all: women of a certain age, women with a uterus, women without reproductive health complications, women who are not pregnant or, often, breast-feeding. The Moon is there for all of us, all the time. Is that not a powerful concept? In this chaotic world, with so much difference and sadness and love, we are all unified together on the same globe, under the same sky, able to see the same Moon.

Can you imagine how powerful it would be if we all worked with the Moon together, at the same time? This practice connects us to something bigger, and that is a great starting point to foster the spirit of genuine connection with each other, seeing points of unity in and among our diversity. The ultimate sameness is that we are all alive on *this* planet, having our highly individualized experiences on

Earth. This is duality and oneness, held together in a beautiful paradox.

Plants begin to break down at this time, highlighting the remnants of beauty that remain. In the seasonal cycle, this is the period marked by the autumnal or fall equinox; energized by midnight in the night cycle, this is also the period in our life cycle where we transition to old age. It is a time when we have much to share and the Yang energy that motivates us to share it.[69]

The focal point for this Moon phase, then, is: **The concept of giving back.**

Up until this point, the journey through the Moon cycle has been one of self-knowledge and inquiry. A journey of self-discovery and delight in the abundance that flows when we clarify, nurture, and take action on our intentions and goals.

Our practice up to this point has emphasized our own personal development, but we cannot forget the element of collaboration and connection under the Moon. If we see the Moon as representing the feminine part of self, we must also remember these feminine qualities of relating to and seeing ourselves as part of a greater whole, rather than focusing solely on our inner journey.

You do not need to feel guilty about paying attention to the self. If we are lucky enough to be in a situation where we can allocate resources, time, attention, and energy to the improvement of the self, then we should *Know thyself*, so we can act accordingly. Nonetheless, personal empowerment is not the final goal of this particular lunar practice.

We may be here on Earth to grow, but we are not here to grow alone. What is the point of personal development, of cultivation? Yes, we want to enjoy the process and the journey, but that cannot be the end of the story. Moving beyond the self to making a difference in the world is a characteristic of most of the wonderful, intelligent, and privileged people I have encountered in a variety of university and corporate workplaces. They devote themselves to making a discernible positive impact on the world through government, research, service, and nonprofit work. Those who are out there making a difference have mastered their craft, and they are not always talking about it.

The point is that once you have empowered yourself, giving back to others around you is a natural next step. Simply doing well yourself has a ripple effect in, well, everything that you do and all that you are has a ripple effect. With care and intention, your ripple effect will be positive. However, the point of this phase goes further than just doing well yourself; the widening gap between rich and poor even in developed nations shows that.

Take this Yang phase as an opportunity to actually give back, rather than merely talking about being of service.

TO WHOM WILL YOU GIVE?

The giving-back phase occurs at each of the Moon phases. Of course, this Yang phase, like all the other Moon phases, simply offers a particular focal point, a useful lens; you can give back at any time throughout the Moon cycle.

The point is to give back in your own unique way. Giving back involves more than just radiating outward, as if you were a lily—it involves effort and practical action. This is a Yang phase, after all.

However, cast your mind back to the less effective ways to be Yang that were outlined in an earlier chapter. If you find that you are exhausted or depleted by giving back, then it may be worthwhile to consider whether you are giving at the expense of yourself. Giving or serving without boundaries can lead to self-sacrifice, and that is not the type of giving that is productive on an ongoing basis. Why? You will burn out eventually, meaning that you will not be able to serve at all. In fact, you will need others to take care of you.

Give back in your own unique way.

The women who tend to be drawn to working with me are the ones who are big-hearted and incredibly generous. They have a tendency to overgive at the sacrifice of the self. This chapter is written with these women in mind, and is the reason why giving back is emphasized as the seventh of eight Moon phases—not because giving is not important enough to be featured in the top six, but because you need to fill your own cup so that you can give in a sustainable and high-impact way.

If you find that you are utterly exhausted at this Moon phase, consider: Do you need to give to yourself?

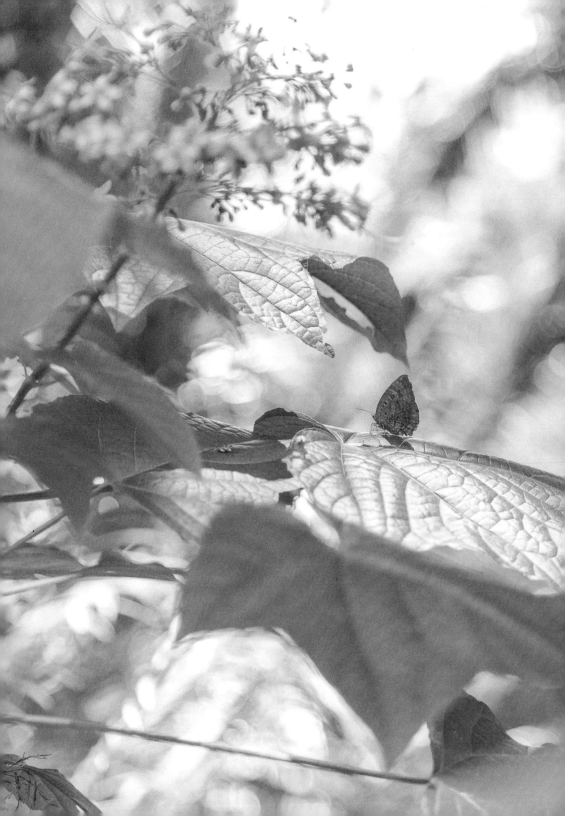

We may be here on Earth to *grow,* but we are not here to *grow alone.*

This may be you if you are the mother of small children, if you are the caregiver for elderly parents, or if you are in a tough job in the service industry. There are many other examples. If this is you: Can you find the small ways that you can fill up your cup in this phase?

GIVE FROM A PLACE OF ABUNDANCE

High-impact, effective, and sustainable giving comes from a place of abundance. This means that you *know* that there is enough for you; this ensures that you are able to give joyously from the overflow of what you have. Indeed, abundant giving comes naturally when you are in the flow, and you feel compelled and delighted to keep your gifts flowing—not out of guilt or some other heavy burden but because it is in the natural order of things for you to share what you have.

And no, abundant giving does not need to break the bank. Some ideas for giving at this Moon phase:

> **Did you feel grateful** for someone's words or actions (now or at a previous time) during the previous Moon phase? Could you reach out now with a heartfelt, handwritten thank-you note—even if you don't know the person?

> **Do you have a friend**, family member, neighbor, or community member in need? Could you bring her food or offer to look after her kids? Could you feed her dog or offer your help in some other practical way?

❭ **Could you make** a weekly or monthly ongoing commitment to volunteer at a local nonprofit? You could even find a way that you could help a charity remotely via the Internet.

❭ **Could you write** a letter to a local politician, or make a submission to a government body that speaks to an important issue? You may be surprised at how much of an impact this can have—and where power is actually located (a hint: it might not be on your Facebook newsfeed).

❭ **Could you extend** a social or dinner invitation to someone who is lonely?

❭ **Could you give** genuine and heartfelt compliments to a friend or colleague, or even to someone you do not know very well?

❭ **Could you give** the gift of time and presence to someone who needs a shoulder to cry on or a sounding board?

❭ **Could you send** flowers to a friend in another town, especially one you haven't spoken with recently?

❭ **Could you create** a freebie or value-add for your clients? Something to say thank you, not a step in a sales sequence.

❭ **Do you have** the capacity to help out a colleague, employee, or employer in a useful way? Could you offer to assist with his work or give him words of encouragement?

❭ **Could you commit** to giving something to charity in the future? Could you make a small donation now?

GIVE WITHOUT STRINGS

Consider avoiding giving because you want to get something in return. When you give, you want to be able to give without strings attached, as subtle as these may be. Recall how icky Jennifer felt in the previous chapter when Jay offered to buy her a coffee. He wanted her to give him her time in return.

If you treat people in a way that is even subtly manipulative, they will feel it. You may end up coercing those with low self-esteem—a messy dynamic. Over time, however, you will repel those with high self-esteem. This type of giving also fractures community, building cynicism and mistrust.

Preventing this kind of giving requires shrewd and sometimes painful observation of yourself, in life and work. Check in with yourself. Ask yourself what is motivating you to give. Is your desire accompanied by a sense of scarcity, of missing out, of needing to get something? Check in with your body. When you give, how does it feel? Expansive and joyful and no-strings-attached, or contracted and tense? The latter is an indication that you may need to consider why you are giving. You need to fill up your own cup and ensure that you are fully nourished first.

If you choose to give to yourself, then do so and enjoy it. If you choose to give to others at this phase, then actually give to others. Giving can and does feel wonderful, but that is a by-product, not the goal. The sole point of giving is not to make yourself feel good. Your altruism isn't directed at you.

When you are choosing to give to others, then give to others. Do it generously and wholeheartedly. Can you imagine what the world would be like if we all gave generously and freely to others, from that place of abundance? Try it and see what happens in your immediate environment.

CONCLUSION

Giving from an abundant place is the key to sustainable, effective, and high-impact giving. The more we are able to give from that place—indeed, the more we give rather than merely thinking or fantasizing, the more we *give* rather than *taking* or tearing down—the more we are able to construct and grow. We actually make the positive impact that we crave. We become a gift to, rather than a burden on, this world.

Giving from an abundant place not only feels good, but it grounds us in real life. It positions us as co-creators and collaborators, it energizes us and positions us to give back in progressively bigger and more meaningful ways. Practicing giving at this Moon phase allows us to do our bit in creating a better life for ourselves, and also to participate in creating healthy families and communities.

At this time of change and instability on the planet, we need to give. At a time of growing inequality, when we have the opportunity, we need to give. Giving from a pure expression of an expanding heart, giving because we want to share both our unique and our beautifully normal gifts, giving without expectation of return: this is an expression of our humanity.

Summary

❭ The focal point for this Moon phase is the concept of giving back. This phase reminds us that we cannot forget the element of collaboration and connection under the one Moon. This Moon phase is for seeing ourselves as part of a great whole here on Earth.

❭ Take the opportunity in this Yang phase to actually give back, as opposed to just thinking or fantasizing about doing it. However, abundant giving does not need to involve lavish gestures or break the bank. You can give a compliment, a flower, or practical help. When you choose to give to others, do so generously and wholeheartedly.

❭ Consider whether you are giving at the expense of yourself; giving without boundaries can lead to self-sacrifice. Fill up your own cup so that you can give in a sustainable and high-impact way.

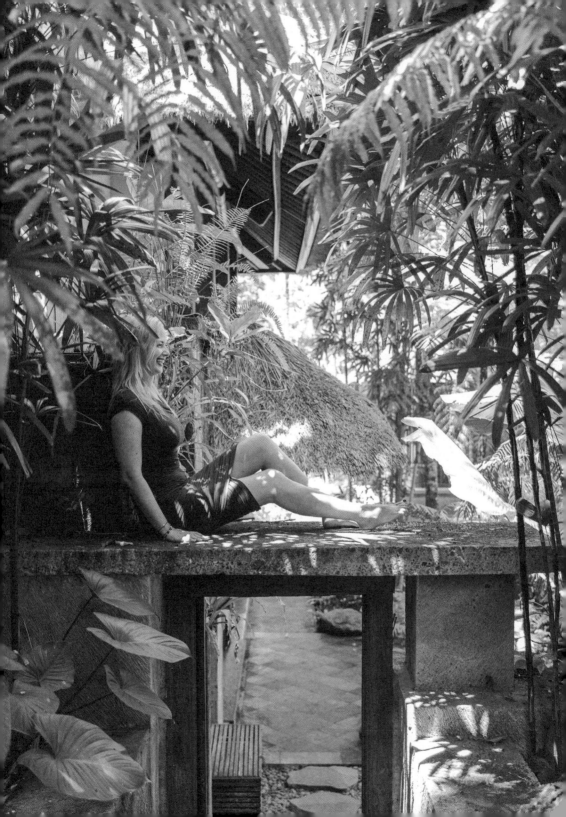

There are times to cultivate and create,
when you nurture your world and give
birth to new ideas and ventures.

There are times of flourishing and abundance,
when life feels in full bloom, energized and expanding.

And there are times of fruition,
when things come to an end.
They have reached their climax and must
be harvested before they begin to fade.

And finally, of course, there are times that are cold,
and cutting and empty, times when the spring
of new beginnings seems like a distant dream.

Those rhythms in life are natural events.
They weave into one another as day follows night,
bringing, not messages of hope and fear,
but messages of how things are.[70]

—CHÖGYAM TRUNGPA RINPOCHE

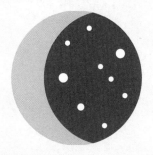

Balsamic Moon

This is the nature of cycles: ebb and flow. The peak and the trough. The darkness and the light. Ascent and descent.

During the Balsamic Moon phase, the Moon returns to darkness. It lasts for some days, until the Moon cycle begins again with the next New Moon. In plant cycles, this is the time of dying back; it also corresponds with the darkest time of winter and those notoriously difficult hours before sunrise (we have all convinced ourselves of all the world's woes while lying awake at 3 a.m.). It also represents the weeks before our birthday, the bleed in our menstrual cycle, and the time of old age in the life cycle. This latter is of course the time of our greatest wisdom and of the collection of knowledge from our life.[71] The crone was once one of the most valued people in society, worthy of the greatest respect and honor: she was not packed off to the nursing home.

The Balsamic Moon phase can be one of the most challenging phases to navigate. In the entirety of this lunar practice, I work with this Moon phase in a metaphorical way. It is not much of a stretch of the imagination to see that when we pause in the final Yin phase, we are brought face-to-face with the subconscious anxiety associated with the ultimate transformation: death.

Of course, many of us are terrified of death. We tend to ignore the great taboo altogether—an understandable fear for a single-life worldview. Of course, death can be metaphorical as well, marking the end point of one chapter before the next begins—a consolation familiar to anyone who has drawn the Death card in tarot. In *Mysteries of the Dark Moon*, Demetra George writes that:

> *Because our perceptions of the dark are filled with images of loss, pain, and suffering, we react with fear, panic, anxiety, confusion, depression and desperation whenever we go through the many dark phase periods in our lives. Often what we have known in the past no longer exists, and what is yet to come has not yet appeared.*[72]

If we work with the Yin and the Yang throughout the Moon cycle—and especially during with this Moon phase, the *most* Yin of all the Yin phases (recall here the concept of relativity between Yin and Yang)—we can practice in a gentle and safe way the inhabiting of the in-between. Then we are not rattled when a bigger transition comes to pass, such as the inevitable finishing of projects and chapters of life, or the parting of ways with someone close to us through death, divorce, or any other form of ultimate ending.

To align with cycles is to open to the reality of what it is to be in the body, on this Earth: the surge of energy and its decline. The building, the shedding, and the growth that comes again. The ovulation, the bleed, the rebuilding. The gestation, the birth. The rise, the fall. The love. The loss. And love, again.

It always starts again.

This is the essence of the cycle. It always winds down to a close, but each ending marks a winding up. This is the substance of abundance: it does not run out. There is always more. There is always another Moon cycle arriving. There is always another New Moon, a slow return of light after the dark Moon reaches its darkest ebb. There is peace and calm in relaxing into this secure order.

How far you extend this metaphor depends on your own belief system about what happens after you shuffle off your mortal coil: I suspect that cycles continue beyond our time on Earth, which in turn gives me comfort about death and dying. This may be an aspect of effective *living*, which is best in the here and now, with our senses active and our human feet on the ground.

Embracing the ever-changing nature of cycles is one way to soothe suffering and to find a sense of peace in your everyday life. There is no "endpoint," no destination branded "happy." There are moments of delight and pain, joy and terror, bliss and agony. There is presence and embodiment in a life fully lived, a life where change is the constant—where the future is bright with potential and a new adventure and opportunity wait just around the corner.

What if these Moon phases do not accord with your own cycles? This is a question I commonly receive. What this practice aims to uncover for you is *self-knowledge*: an awareness of how your body moves, how your energy rises and falls. It is a way for you to appreciate and predict your own ebbs and flows, so you do not stay in the old pattern of push, push, and then collapse. Always honor and elevate the wisdom of your own body above what *anyone* tells you. This practice is offered to you as a guide: an invitation to move beyond literal and rigid interpretations, to stop trying to be perfect, quit fretting about whether you are doing it "right," and listen to and trust your own inner knowing above all else.

Always honor and elevate the wisdom of your own body above what anyone tells you.

WHAT IS THE VALUE OF THE MOON, THEN?

I work with the Moon as a mirror. When I look up at night (or day) and see the Moon, she reminds me to come within, check in with my body, my feelings, my emotional world, even just for a minute. I still need reminding to come back to base.

She is my natural anchor.

When I see the Moon,
she reminds me to
come within, check in
with my body, my feelings,
my emotional world,
even just for a minute.

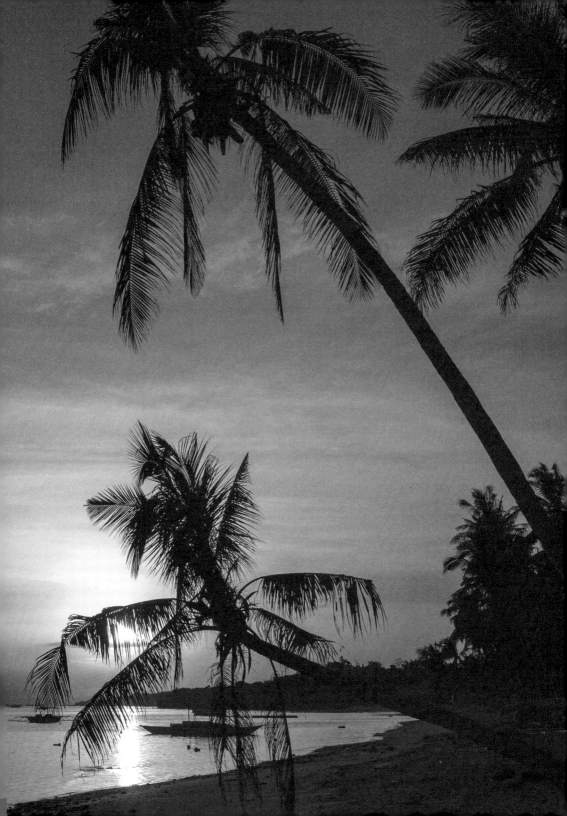

The Moon also calms me. In moments when I start to worry that there is not enough for me, when I fall into lack, I remember what rich soil there is in my life, and that I may take action to intentionally and consciously till the ground.

She is my gentle guide into the mystery.

The Moon's Yin and Yang phases also remind me to keep embedding the principles of intentional rest into my life. I know that I am healthier, more *well*, when I pay attention to my well-being—even for brief glimpses.

She is my natural timekeeper.

SET UP YOUR SUCCESS

You can do this in a random way (which is fine), but you can also set aside time for unstructured play.

Schedule time in your diary or calendar at some point during a Balsamic Moon phase to just *be*. Embed this in your life. If you do not have vast amounts of time, that is fine. You can still make it work; everything is relative, right? Turn off your Wi-Fi and phone, and you might find more time.

Schedule even half an hour of *being* time. Or fifteen minutes. Whatever you can find. Actually schedule it in your calendar: set up the structure to hold your flow.

Now, that doesn't include scrolling through social media, or drinking wine, or watching Netflix—that is distraction time (which I also encourage, but in its right place!).

This right here is *being* time.

How often do we not realize how tired we really are until we stop?

Embedding the "pause" in our lives is one way to listen and honor this.

HOW TO BE?

If *being* is really uncomfortable for you, know that you are not alone. This is one of the most challenging aspects of unwinding, this go-go-go that modern Western culture expects. Know that this will become easier with practice, so allow yourself to practice in low-risk environments.

> **Go for a walk**—not to lose weight, or get fit, or get the kids out of the house, or to blow off steam, or to replay the conversation with your mother. Just to walk.

> **Go to a café** without your phone, laptop, or other external distractions. Don't go to think. Go to savor your coffee or chai. Go to feel the Sun on your face.

> **On a busy day at work,** go to the bathroom. Put the lid down, sit down, shut your eyes, and just breathe for a few minutes. This is *so basic*, but it can help you navigate a stressful day or afternoon (I know—I've been there, over and over).

> **Make love.** To yourself, or with someone else.

> **Meditate.** Set up a corner in your home, light a candle, find a patch of Sun, or join a meditation group. Or go outside. Find a labyrinth to walk. A nice path will also work. Don't meditate to get enlightened. Meditate to experience what it is to be you.

> **Play with your kids**—or your sister's kids (or someone else near to you). Failing that, a puppy. Don't play because you are aiming to awaken the creative sense within you. Play to play.

> **Meet up with someone you love.** No phone, no agenda. No checking off all the boxes in life, or gossiping about your mutual problematic friend. Just be together.

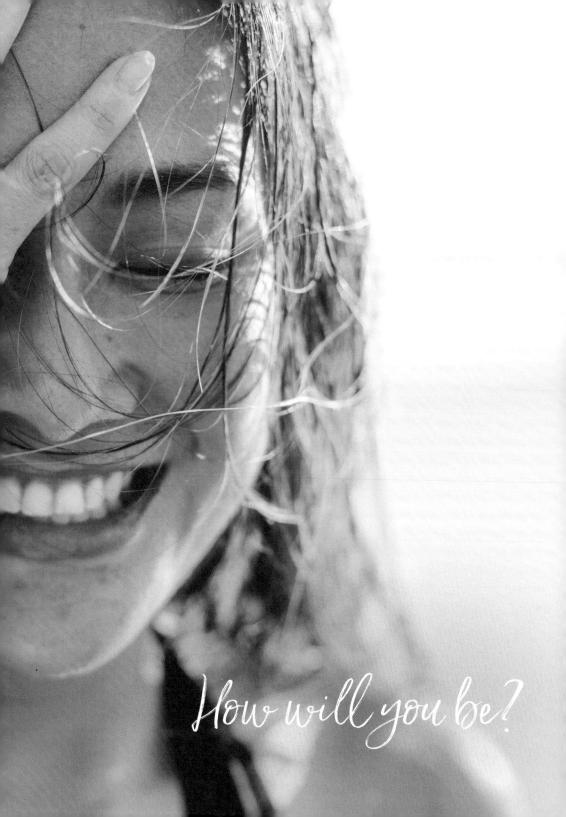

How will you be?

Ditch the goals and the outcomes.

Allow yourself to laugh.

Allow yourself to rest.

Allow yourself to be.

This is where the magic happens. When will you schedule the time to just *be* during this Moon phase?

REFLECTION

The "New!" and "Improved!" labels are used in sales and marketing for a reason: we humans seem to be eager to leap to the next thing.

One of the essential principles of this practice, though, is to finish what you start. There is no need to rush onto the next thing without reflecting on where we have been, where we are, and what has brought us to this place.

Because life has a habit of showing up for us, we sometimes do not even realize what we have learned about ourselves, or what has enriched our lives, until we take the time to pause and reflect. We have to take time to acknowledge this, and to feel grateful.

I encourage you to reflect on your practice each day, but set aside some specific time during this Moon phase to reflect on the entire cycle.

Allow your reflections to shape your next New Moon intention.

Reflect now:

❭ What have you learned about yourself in this Moon cycle?

❯ What surprised you about this process?

_____
_____
_____
_____
_____

❯ What will you do differently next time?

_____
_____
_____
_____
_____

❯ What has come into your life as you practice the exercises in this book?

_____
_____
_____
_____
_____

❯ What might be the contours of your next New Moon intention?

_____
_____
_____
_____
_____

For there is, of course, another Moon cycle coming.

As you tilt your chin to the sky to see the light emerge, rub your toes on the ground and feel your body.

Once you have tapped into your inner well of strength and power,

Once you have found the courage to enter the crevices of your heart and soul,

Once you have been brave enough to love and roll in ecstasy with what you find,

Once you bloom into the magnificence of who you are, and once you ride the rhythms of nature in tune with yourself,

This is when you are alive.

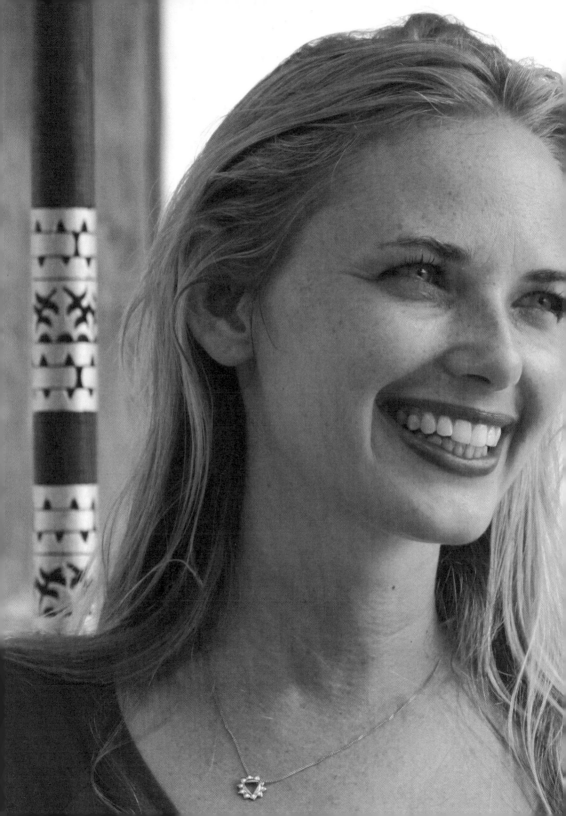

Now that you have

*followed
the Moon cycle,*

it's time to

begin again …

Stay Connected

LUNAR ABUNDANCE WEBSITE

Visit my website www.LunarAbundance.com for free graphics and audio resources about this lunar practice, download your free lunar planner with the dates of all eight Moon phases for the year, and sign up for free e-letters that will remind you of the time and date of each upcoming New and Full Moon. You will also find journaling resources to help you develop your practice.

LUNAR ABUNDANCE SALON

Join the Lunar Abundance Salon, an online program where we delve much deeper into this practice by following the Moon for a full solar year, working with several specific intention themes and aspects of abundance.

SOCIAL MEDIA

Come and say hi to me on social media, and share your experiences (I love to hear from you!):

Instagram @ezziespencer
Facebook @ezziespencer

Acknowledgments

I have been lucky to have wonderful teachers and guides who have helped shape my ideas, many of whom are listed in the following Resources section. Steven Forrest and Demetra George, Kevin Farrow, Saida Désilets, Marc Laurenson and Tom Starke have been key—and, of course, I have been anchored and guided by La Luna herself.

There were so many helpers for this actual book. Rachel MacDonald activated the project by persuading me to write this book in 2013, and then provided characteristically insightful comments on the beta chapters during the eventual writing phase. The original book outline emerged during Tara Bliss's writing workshop in 2015. Esmé Weijan Wang was an exemplary and caring editor in 2016. Alice Grundy at Xoum Publishing arrived at the perfect time, elevating this project to another level. Bronwyn Stange gave invaluable research assistance.

The US edition would not have materialized without the belief of my dream literary agent, Meg Thompson, and perfect editor, Cindy De La Hoz, at Running Press.

Many more have supported the project, in practical and magical ways—Amber Rae, Andrew Moon, Kerry Rowett, Cassandra Hawkins, Kate Erlenbusch, Sarah Gleeson, Julie Parker, Megan Dalla-Camina, Kate Reardon, Louise Robinson, Jen Blackstock, Theresa Reed, and Elle Luna have all played parts. Pamela

Mattson inspired the tables about more and less effective Yin and Yang. Emma Kate Codrington and Andrew Moon took many of the beautiful photographs in this book at Villa Beji Indah and Trinity Gardens in Bali.

The book could not have been birthed without the perpetual energetic support of family: my mother, father, brother, and sister, always present. Many dear girlfriends have also jived with it: Kate, Katarina, Jess, Alex, Frances, Michelle, Erin, Nassim, Sarah, Emily, Louise, Rachael, Zoe, Amanda, Azita, Barb, Amber, Bec, Cassie, Pernilla, Moa, and Mayet—thanks for the chats, laughs, and support!

The rich island of Bali has held me through much the writing phase—with some pivotal moments in Gertrude & Alice at Bondi, too (thank you, Jane Turner). The creation months were charmed at Villa Beji Indah (Timmy, I am eternally grateful) and in the bosom of Trinity Gardens with Susanna Nova.

Of course, my Lunar Abundance Salon Sisters have supported me from the get-go—these women, my private clients, and those who read my blog, e-letters, and online writings have enriched this work through questions, comments, and commitment to what is a living, breathing, and ever-expanding practice.

With love and gratitude—thank you.

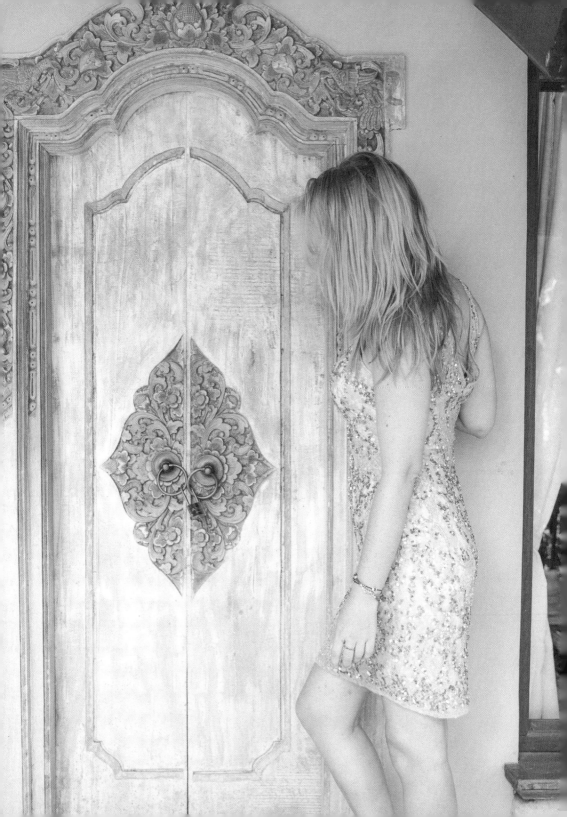

The habit of writing . . . for my own eye
only is good practice. It loosens the ligaments.
Never mind the misses and the stumbles.[73]

—VIRGINIA WOOLF

A Note on Notes

As you read this book, I encourage you to respond with your own thoughts and feelings.

Here is some room to engage further, to try things out and to experiment. Enjoy the process and remember that the practice is ongoing and that each cycle offers a new opportunity to explore further.

Notes

Notes

Notes

Notes

Notes

Notes

Notes

Notes

Notes

Notes

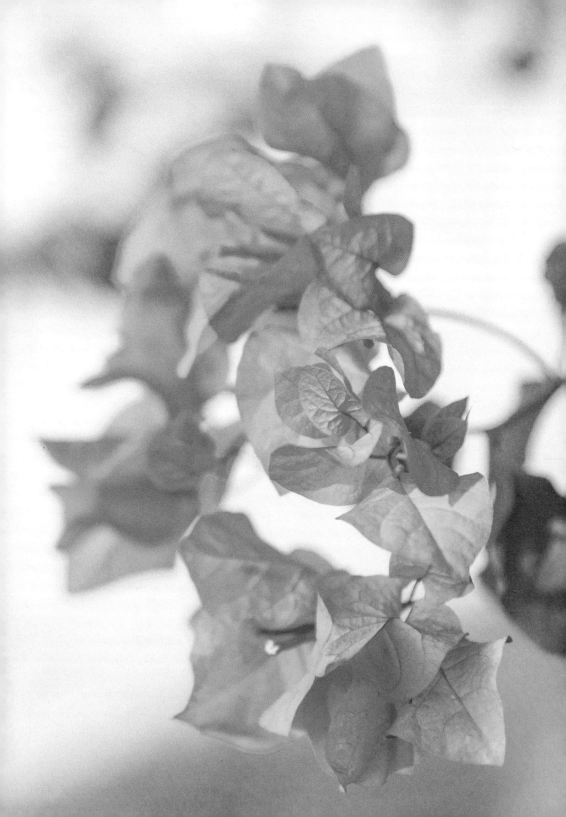

Resources

GODDESSES, MYTHOLOGY, AND ARCHETYPES

M. J. Abadie, *The Goddess in Every Girl: Develop Your Feminine Power* (Simon Pulse/Beyond Words, 2013).

David Adams Leeming, *Creation Myths of the World: Parts I–II*, 2nd ed. (ABC-CLIO, 2009).

David Adams Leeming and Jake Page, *Myths of the Female Divine* (Oxford University Press, 1996).

Rachel Alexander, *Myths, Symbols and Legends of Solar System Bodies* (Springer, 2015).

Lasara Firefox Allen, *Jailbreaking the Goddess: A Radical Revisioning of Feminist Spirituality* (Llewellyn, 2016).

Tamra Andrews, *Dictionary of Nature Myths: Legends of the Earth, Sea, and Sky* (Oxford University Press, 2000).

Raj Arumugam, *Ganesha, Laksmi and Saraswati* (TTS, 2006).

Jane Caputi, *Goddesses and Monsters: Women, Myth, Power and Popular Culture* (University of Wisconsin Press, 2004).

Charles Russell Coulter and Patricia Turner, *Encyclopedia of Ancient Deities* (Mcfarland, 2012).

Donna Cunningham, *The Moon in Your Life: Being a Lunar Type in a Solar World* (Weiser Books, 1996).

Christine DeVine and Marie Hendry (eds.), *Turning Points and Transformations: Essays on Language, Literature and Culture* (Cambridge Scholars Publishing, 2011).

Frances Devlin-Glass and Lyn McCredden (eds.), *Feminist Poetics of the Sacred: Creative Suspicions* (Oxford University Press, 2001).

Demetra George, *Mysteries of the Dark Moon: The Healing Power of the Dark Goddess* (HarperCollins, 1992).

Helena Goscilo, Martin Skoro, and Jack Zipes, *Baba Yaga: The Wild Witch of the East in Russian Fairy Tales*, translated by Sibelan Forrester (University Press of Mississippi, 2013).

Timothy Harley, *Moon Lore* (CreateSpace, 2015).

Lisa Hunt, *Celestial Goddesses: An Illustrated Meditation Guide* (Llewellyn Publications, 2001).

Alice Karlsdóttir, *Norse Goddess Magic: Trancework, Mythology, and Ritual* (Destiny Books, 2015).

William Klauser, *The Esoteric Codex: Deities of the Underworld* (Lulu, 2015).

C. Scott Littleton (ed.), *Gods, Goddesses, and Mythology*, vol. 4 (Marshall Cavendish, 2005).

Edain McCoy, *Magick & Rituals of the Moon* (Llewellyn Publications, 2001).

Nemi Sharan Mittal, *World-Famous Mythologies* (Pustak Mahal, 2010).

J. Mohapatra, *Wellness in Indian Festivals and Rituals* (PartridgeIndia, 2013).

Patricia Monaghan, *Encyclopedia of Goddesses and Heroines* (Greenwood, 2009).

Jim Ollhoff, *Japanese Mythology* (ABDO and Daughters, 2011).

Tracy Pintchman (ed.), *Women's Lives, Women's Rituals in the Hindu Tradition* (Oxford University Press, 2007).

Pat Remler, *Egyptian Mythology, A to Z* 3rd ed. (Chelsea House Publications, 2010).

Anita Ryan, *Moon Goddess: Manifest Your Dreams* (Lulu, 2008).

Daniela Schenker, *Kuan Yin: Accessing the Power of the Divine Feminine* (Sounds True, 2007).

Karen Tate, *Sacred Places of Goddess: 108 Destinations* (CC Publishing, 2006).

Marion Woodman and Elinor Dickson, *Dancing in the Flames: The Dark Goddess in the Transformation of Consciousness* (Shambhala, 1997).

Jennifer Barker Woolger and Roger J. Woolger, *The Goddess Within: A Guide to the Eternal Myths That Shape Women's Lives* (Ballantine Books, 1987).

MENSTRUAL CYCLES

Claire Baker, *Adore Your Cycle: Find Your Flow, Work Your Menstrual Magic and Change the Way You Live Your Life* (2016).

Chris Bobel, *New Blood: Third-Wave Feminism and the Politics of Menstruation* (Rutgers University Press, 2010).

Roni Edlund, Damo Mitchell, and Sophie Johnson, *Daoist Nei Gong for Women: The Art of the Lotus and the Moon* (Singing Dragon, 2016).

Lisa Fazio, *Sacred Lunation: Rhythms for the Feminine Cycle* (Hawthorne Hill Herbs, 2016).

Judy Grahn, *Blood, Bread, and Roses: How Menstruation Created the World* (Beacon Press, 1993).

Miranda Gray, *Red Moon* (FastPrint, 2009).

Miranda Gray, *The Optimized Woman: If You Want to Get Ahead, Get a Cycle* (O Books, 2009).

Barbara Hanneloré and Naomi Rose, *The Moon and You: A Woman's Guide to an Easier Monthly Cycle* (Bell House, 2014).

Rachael Hertogs, *Thirteen Moons*, 2nd ed. (Lulu, 2011).

DeAnna L'am, *Becoming Peers: Mentoring Girls into Womanhood* (Red Moon Publishing, 2007).

Lisa Lister and Meggan Watterson, *Code Red: Know Your Flow, Unlock Your Super Powers and Create a Bloody Amazing Life. Period* (SHE Press UK, 2015).

Martha K. McClintock, "Menstrual Synchrony and Suppression," 299 (1971) *Nature*: 244–245.

Martha K. McClintock, "On the Nature of Mammalian and Human Pheromones," *Annals of the New York Academy of Sciences* 855 (1998): 390–392.

Rachel Kauder Nalebuff, *My Little Red Book* (Twelve, 2009).

Lucy H. Pearce, *Reaching for the Moon* (Createspace, 2013).

Lucy H. Pearce, *Moon Time: Harness the Ever-Changing Energy of Your Menstrual Cycle*, 2nd ed. (Womancraft Publishing, 2015).

Linda Sparrowe, *Yoga for a Healthy Menstrual Cycle* (Shambhala, 2004).

Cassie Premo Steele, *Moon Days: Creative Writings about Menstruation* (Summerhouse Press, 1999).

Kisma K. Stepanich, *Sister Moon Lodge: The Power and Mystery of Menstruation* (Llewellyn Publications, 1992).

Alisa Vitti, *WomanCode: Perfect Your Cycle, Amplify Your Fertility, Supercharge Your Sex Drive, and Become a Power Source* (HarperOne, 2014).

Linda Heron Wind, *New Moon Rising: Reclaiming the Sacred Rites of Menstruation* (Heron Press, 2014).

LUNAR CYCLES AND RESEARCH

Leonie A. Calver, Barrie J. Stokes, and Geoffrey K. Ibister, "The Dark Side of the Moon," *Australian Medical Journal*, 191, nos. 11–12 (2009): 692–694.

Cristy Gelling, "Full Moon May Mean Less Sleep: Slumber Waxes and Wanes with Lunar Cycles," *Society for Science and the Public*, 184, no. 4 (2013): 15.

S. L. Gray and R. G. Harrison, "Diagnosing Eclipse-Induced Wind Change," *Proceedings of the Royal Society*, 468 (2012): 1839–1850.

Sandra and David Mosley, *Zodiac Arts*, http://zodiacarts.com.

Ernest Naylor, *Moonstruck: How Lunar Cycles Affect Life* (Oxford University Press, 2015).

Richard D. Neal and Malcolm Colledge, "The Effect of the Full Moon on General Practice Consultation Rates," *Family Practice*, 17, no. 6 (2000): 472–474.

Jack R. Pyle and Taylor Reese, *Raising with the Moon: The Complete Guide to Gardening and Living by the Signs of the Moon* (Parkway Publishers, 2003).

Dane Rudhyar, *The Lunation Cycle* (Llewellyn Publications, 1967).

Clive L. N. Ruggles, *Ancient Astronomy: An Encyclopedia of Cosmologies and Myth* (ABC-CLIO, 2005).

Michael Smithe, Ilona Croy, and Kerstin Persson Waye, "Human Sleep and Cortical Reactivity Are Influenced by Lunar Phase", *Current Biology*, 24, no. 12 (2014): R551–R552.

Rudolf Steiner, *Agriculture Course: The Birth of the Biodynamic Method*, translated by George Adams (Rudolf Steiner Press, 2014).

C. P. Thakur and Dilip Sharma, "Full Moon and Crime," *British Medical Journal*, 289 no. 6460 (1984): 789–1791.

David Whitehouse, *The Moon: A Biography* (Headline Book Publishing, 2001).

CYCLES—OTHER

Edward Dewey and Edwin Dakin, *Cycles: The Science of Prediction* (Holt and Company, 1947).

George Haralambie, "The Global Crisis and Cyclical Theory," *Theoretical and Applied Economics*, 11, no. 564 (2011): 79–88.

Rebecca Orleane, *The Return of the Feminine: Honoring the Cycles of Nature* (AuthorHouse, 2010).

BODY LOVE, SEXUALITY, AND ESTEEM

Saida Desilets, *The Emergence of the Sensual Woman—Awakening Our Erotic Innocence* (2005).

Tracy Gaudet and Paula Spencer, *Consciously Female: How to Listen to Your Body and Your Soul for a Lifetime of Healthier Living* (Bantam, 2004).

Anita Johnston, *Eating in the Light of the Moon: How Women Can Transform Their Relationships with Food Through Myths, Metaphors and Storytelling* (Gürze Books, 2000).

Azita Nahai, *From Trauma to Dharma* (Forthcoming, 2018).

Christiane Northrup, *Women's Bodies, Women's Wisdom* (Piatkus Books, 1995).

SELECTED SPIRITUALITY, JUNGIAN, AND DEPTH PSYCHOLOGY

Sera Beak, *Red Hot and Holy: A Heretic's Love Story* (Sounds True, 2013).

Tara Brach, *Radical Acceptance: Embracing Your Life with the Heart of a Buddha* (Bantam, 2004).

Tara Brach, *True Refuge: Finding Peace and Freedom in Your Own Awakened Heart* (Bantam, 2016).

Mariana Caplan, *Eyes Wide Open: Cultivating Discernment on the Spiritual Path* (Sounds True, 2009).

Pema Chodron, *Living Beautifully: With Uncertainty and Change* (Shambhala Publications, 2012).

Thomas Cleary (ed. and trans.), *Immortal Sisters: Secret Teachings of Taoist Women* (North Atlantic Books, 1996).

Thomas Cleary (ed. and trans.), *Secret of the Golden Flower* (HarperCollins, 1993).

Thomas Cleary and Sartaz Aziz, *Twilight Goddess: Spiritual Feminism and Feminine Spirituality* (Shambhala Press, 2000).

Rose Mary Dougherty, *Discernment: A Path to Spiritual Awakening* (Paulist Press, 2009).

Judith Duerk, *Circle of Stones: Woman's Journey to Herself*, 10th anniversary ed. (New World Library, 2004).

Dr. Clarissa Pinkola Estés, *Women Who Run with the Wolves: Myths and Stories of the Wild Woman Archetype*, reprint ed. (Ballantine Books, 1996).

Kevin Farrow, *The Psychology of the Body* (AcuEnergetics Pty Ltd., 2007).

Kevin Farrow, *Meditation as Medicine* (AcuEnergetics Pty Ltd., 2010).

Kevin Farrow, *Enlighten: Practices for the Modern Mystic* (AcuEnergetics Pty Ltd., 2015).

Jentezen Franklin, *The Amazing Discernment of Women* (Nelson Books, 2006).

Dr. Carl Jung, *Collected Works* (Bollingen Foundation, 1993 [1952]).

Byron Katie, *Loving What Is: Four Questions That Can Change Your Life* (Three Rivers Press, 2003).

Byron Katie, *A Thousand Names for Joy: Living in Harmony with the Way Things Are* (Harmony, 2008).

Tami Lynn Kent, *Wild Feminine: Finding Power, Spirit & Joy in the Female Body* (Atria Books/Beyond Words, 2011).

Robert Augustus Masters, *Spiritual Bypassing: When Spirituality Disconnects Us from What Really Matters* (North Atlantic Books, 2010).

Maureen Murdock, *The Heroine's Journey* (Shambhala, 1990).

Rinpoche Dzogchen Ponlop, *Rebel Buddha: On the Road to Freedom* (Shambhala, 2011).

Barbara Schmidt, *The Practice: Simple Tools for Managing Stress, Finding Inner Peace, and Uncovering Happiness* (Health Communications, Inc., 2014).

Tosha Silver, *Outrageous Openness: Letting the Divine Take the Lead* (Atria Books, 2014).

Krista Tippett, *Becoming Wise: An Inquiry into the Mystery and Art of Living* (Penguin Books, 2016).

FEMINISM

Judith Butler, *Gender Trouble: Feminism and the Subversion of Identity* (Routledge, 2006).

Annabel Crabb, *The Wife Drought* (Ebury Australia, 2014).

Kimberle Crenshaw, *On Intersectionality: The Essential Writings of Kimberle Crenshaw* (Perseus Distribution Services, 2012).

Simone De Beauvoir, *The Second Sex*, translated by Constance Borde and Sheila Malovany-Chevallier) Vintage, 2011).

Germaine Greer, *The Female Eunuch* (Farrar, Straus and Giroux, 2002).

bell hooks, *Feminism Is for Everybody: Passionate Politics* (South End Press, 2000).

Audre Lorde, *Sister Outsider* (Crossing Press, 1984).

Caitlin Moran, *How to Be a Woman* (Ebury Press, 2011).

Susie Orbach, *Fat Is a Feminist Issue* (Arrow Books, 1978).

Brigid Schulte, *Overwhelmed: Work, Love, and Play When No One Has the Time* (Sarah Crichton Books, 2014).

Natasha Walter, *The Return of Sexism* (Virago Press, 2008).

Naomi Wolf, *The Beauty Myth: How Images of Beauty Are Used Against Women* (Harper Perennial, 2002).

Mary Wollstonecraft, *A Vindication of the Rights of Woman*.

PERSONAL DEVELOPMENT, PRODUCTIVITY, AND LEADERSHIP

Dr. Brené Brown, *The Gifts of Imperfection: Let Go of Who You Think You're Supposed to Be and Embrace Who You Are* (Hazelden, 2010).

Dr. Brené Brown, *Rising Strong* (Random House, 2015).

P. R. Clance, and S. A. Imes, "The Impostor Phenomenon in High Achieving Women: Dynamics and Therapeutic Intervention," *Psychotherapy: Theory, Research, and Practice*, 15, no. 3 (1978): 241–247.

Amy Cuddy, *Presence* (Little, Brown and Company, 2015).

Megan Dalla-Camina and Michelle McQuaid, *Lead Like a Woman: Your Essential Guide for True Confidence, Career Clarity, Vibrant Wellbeing and Leadership Success* (Lead Like A Woman Pty Ltd., 2016).

John Gerzema and Michael D'Antonio, *The Athena Doctrine: How Women (and the Men Who Think Like Them) Will Rule the Future* (Jossey-Bass, 2013).

Adam Grant, *Give and Take: A Revolutionary Approach to Success* (Penguin Books, 2014).

Greg McKeown, *Essentialism: The Disciplined Pursuit of Less* (Crown Business, 2014).

POWER OF REST, RELAXATION, AND BREATH

Ericsson, K. Anders, Ralf T. Krampe, and Clemens Tesch-Römer, "The Role of Deliberate Practice in the Acquisition of Expert Performance," *Psychological Review*, 100, no. 3 (1993): 363–406.

Benjamin Baird, Jonathan Smallwood, Michael D. Mrazek, Julia W. Y. Kam, Michael S. Franklin, and Jonathan W. Schooler, "Inspired by Distraction: Mind

 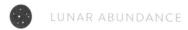

Wandering Facilitates Creative Incubation," *Psychological Science*, 23, no. 10 (2010): 1117–1122.

Volker Busch, Walter Magerl, Uwe Kern, Joachim Haas, Göran Hajak, and Peter Eichhammer, "The Effect of Deep and Slow Breathing on Pain Perception, Autonomic Activity, and Mood Processing—An Experimental Study," *The American Academy of Pain Medicine*, 13, no. 2 (2011): 215–228.

Ap Dijksterhuis, Maarten W. Bos, Loran F. Nordgren, and Rick B. van Baaren, "On Making the Right Choice: The Deliberation-without-Attention Effect," *Science* 311, no. 5763 (2006): 1005–1007.

Mary Helen Immordino-Yang, Joanna A. Christodoulou, and Vanessa Singh, "Rest Is Not Idleness: Implications of the Brain's Default Mode for Human Development and Education," *Perspectives on Psychological Science*, 7, no. 4 (2012): 352–364.

Ravinder Jerath and Vernon A. Barnes, "Augmentation of Mind-Body Therapy and Role of Deep Slow Breathing," *Journal of Complementary and Integrative Medicine*, 13, no. 2 (2011): 566–571.

Ravinder Jerath, Vernon A. Barnes, Molly W. Crawford, and Kyler Harden, "Self-Regulation of Breathing as a Primary Treatment for Anxiety," *Applied Psychophysiology and Biofeedback*, 40 (2015): 107–11.

Ravinder Jerath, J. W. Edry, Vernon A. Barnes, and Vandna Jerath, "Physiology of Long Pranayamic Breathing: Neural Respiratory Elements May Provide a Mechanism That Explains How Slow Deep Breathing Shifts the Autonomic Nervous System," *Medical Hypotheses*, 67, no. 3 (2006): 566–71.

FEELING AND EXPRESSING EMOTIONS

Benjamin P. Chapman, Kevin Fiscella, Ichiro Kawachi, Paul Duberstein, and Peter Muennig, "Emotion Suppression and Mortality Risk Over a 12-Year Follow-Up," *Journal of Psychosomatic Research*, 75, no. 4 (2013): 381–385.

Gordon L. Flett, Paul L. Hewitt and Marnin J. Heisel, "The Destructiveness of Perfectionism Revisited: Implications For the Assessment of Suicide Risk and the Prevention of Suicide," *Review of General Psychology*, 18, no. 3 (2014): 156–172.

X. D. Martin and M. C. Brennan, "Serotonin in human tears" (1994) 4(3) *European Journal of Ophthalmology*, 159–165.

Judith Orloff, *Emotional Freedom: Liberate Yourself From Negative Emotions and Transform Your Life* (Harmony, 2010).

James W. Pennebaker, *Opening Up: The Healing Power of Expressing Emotions*, 2nd ed. (The Guilford Press, 1990).

Michael Philp, Sarah Egan, and Robert Kane, "Perfectionism, Over Commitment to Work, and Burnout in Employees Seeking Workplace Counselling," *Australian Journal of Psychology*, 64, (2012): 68–74.

Julie Sheldon, *The Blessing of Tears* (Hymns Ancient & Modern Ltd., 2004).

Philip M. Ullrich and Susan K. Lutgendorf, "Journaling About Stressful Events: Effects of Cognitive Processing and Emotional Expression," *Annals of Behavioural Medicine*, 24, no. 3 (2002): 244–250.

Els van der Helm, Ninad Gujar, and Matthew P. Walker, "Sleep Deprivation Impairs the Accurate Recognition of Human Emotions," *Sleep*, 33, no. 3 (2010): 335–342.

Ad Vingerhoets, *Why Only Humans Weep: Unravelling the Mysteries of Tears* (Oxford University Press, 2013).

PSYCHOLOGY AND NEUROPSYCHOLOGY

Norman Doidge, *The Brain that Changes Itself* (Penguin Books, 2008).

James Doty, *Into the Magic Shop*, 2nd ed. (Avery, 2016).

Williams James, *The Principles of Psychology* (Holt, 1890).

Thomas Pink, *The Psychology of Freedom* (Cambridge University Press, 1996).

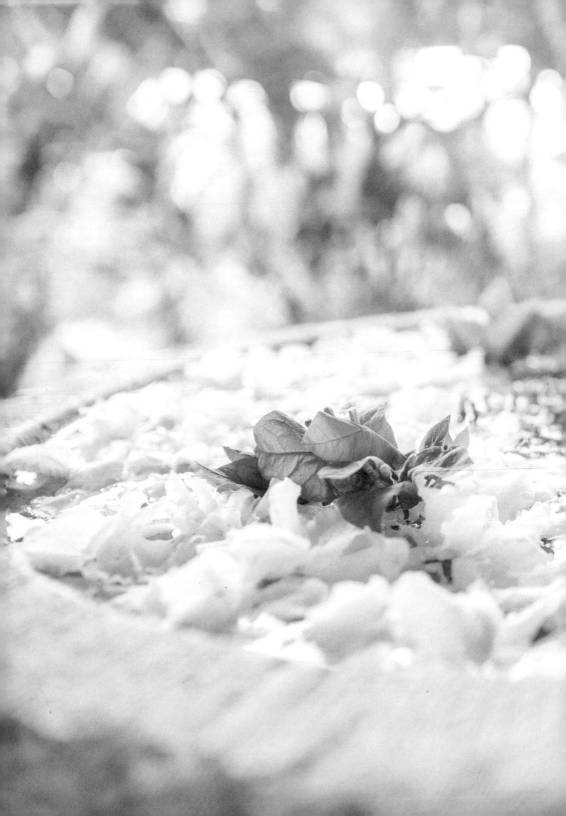

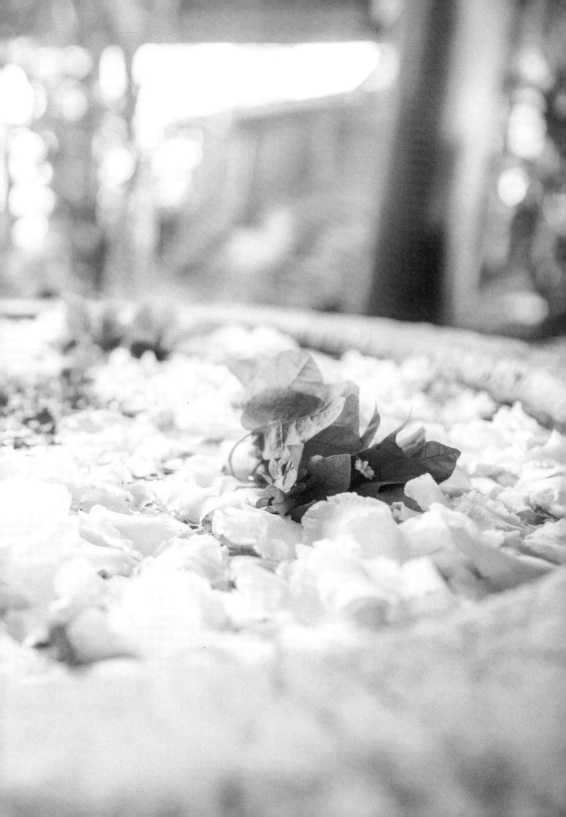

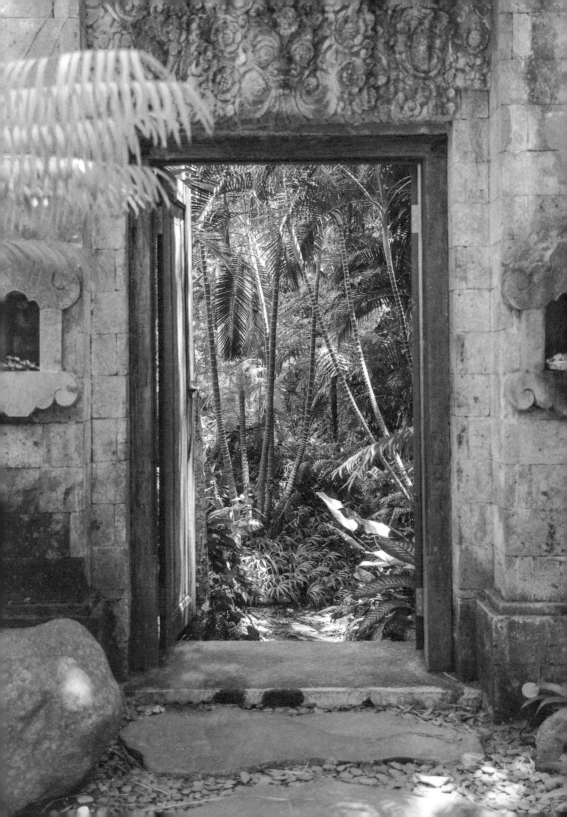

Endnotes

1. Rumi, *The Glance: Songs of Soul Meaning* (Penguin, 2001).

2. Thomas Cleary and Sartaz Aziz, *Twilight Goddess: Spiritual Feminism and Feminine Spirituality* (Shambhala Press, 2000), p. 42.

3. Jane Caputi, *Goddesses and Monsters: Women, Myth, Power and Popular Culture* (University of Wisconsin Press, 2004), p. 328.

4. See Carol Gilligan, *In a Different Voice: Psychological Theory and Women's Development* (Harvard University Press, 1982) and subsequent texts.

5. John Gerzema and Michael D'Antonio, *The Athena Doctrine: How Women (and the Men Who Think Like Them) Will Rule the Future* (Jossey-Bass, 2013); Megan Dalla-Camina and Michelle McQuaid, *Women Who Lead* (Beacon Hill Press, 2016).

6. See Ann Douglas, *The Feminization of American Culture* (Farrar, Straus and Giroux, 1982)—and google this term for numerous hysterical articles.

7. Jeffrey Pfeffer, *Leadership B.S.* (HarperBusiness, 2015).

8. For a much more detailed elucidation on the topic, from a thinker ahead of her time, one who has surely influenced the current rapidly changing public discourse on gender, see Judith Butler, *Gender Trouble* (Routledge, 1992).

9. The original and key text on the concept of intersectionalism—that identities are constructed in multiple ways impacted by gender *and* race and other factors, in combinations that vary in their benefits and disadvantages—see Kimberle Crenshaw, "Mapping the Margins: Intersectionality, Identity Politics, and Violence against Women of Color," *Stanford Law Review* 43, no. 6 (July 1991): 1241–1299.

10. Anne E. Walker, *The Menstrual Cycle* (Routledge, 1997), p. 13.

11. Ernest Naylor, *Moonstruck: How Lunar Cycles Affect Life* (Oxford University Press, 2015), p. 4.

12. Cristy Gelling, "Full Moon May Mean Less Sleep," *Science News* 184, no. 4 (August 24, 2013): 15; C. Cajochen, S. Altanay-Ekici, M. Münch, S. Frey, V. Knoblauch, and A. Wirz-Justice, *Current Biology* 23, no. 15 (August 5, 2013): 1485–1488; "Are Children Like Werewolves? Full Moon and Its Association with Sleep and Activity Behaviors in an International Sample of Children," *Frontiers in Pediatrics* 4 (May 6, 2016). Michael Smithemail, Ilona Croy, and Kerstin Persson Waye, "Human Sleep and Cortical Reactivity Are Influenced by Lunar Phase," 24, issue 12, (June 16, 2014): R551–R552.

13. C. P. Thakur and Dilip Sharma, "Full Moon and Crime," *British Medical Journal* (Clinical Research Edition), 289, no. 6460 (December 22–29, 1984): 1789–1791.

14. Leonie A. Calver, Barrie J. Stokes, and Geoffrey K. Ibister, "The Dark Side of the Moon," *Australian Medical Journal* 191, nos. 11/12 (2009): 692–694; Richard D. Neal and Malcolm Colledge, "The Effect of the Full Moon on General Practice Consultation Rates," *Family Practice* 17, no. 6 (2000): 472–474.

15. Jean-Luc Margot, "No Evidence of Purported Lunar Effect on Hospital Admission Rates or Birth Rates," *Nursing Research* 64, issue 3 (May/June 2015): 168–175.

16. Demetra George, *Mysteries of the Dark Moon: The Healing Power of the Dark Goddess* (HarperCollins, 1992), p. 144.

17. S. L. Gray and R. G. Harrison, "Diagnosing Eclipse-Induced Wind Change," *Proceedings of the Royal Society* 468 (2012): 1839–1850.

18. Dr. Carl Jung, *Synchronicity: An Acausal Connecting Principle* (Bollingen Foundation, 1993 [1952]).

19. A. G. Manning, R. I. Khakimov, R. G. Dall, and A. G. Truscott, "Wheeler's Delayed-Choice Gedanken Experiment with a Single Atom," *Nature Physics* 11 (2015): 539–542. This is explained further in the press release: Australian National University, "Experiment Confirms Quantum Theory Weirdness" (May 27, 2015): www. sciencedaily.com/releases/2015/05/150527103110.htm.

20. Tracy Gaudet and Paula Spencer, *Consciously Female: How to Listen to Your Body and Your Soul for a Lifetime of Healthier Living* (Bantam, 2004). See also Anita Johnston, *Eating in the Light of the Moon: How Women Can Transform Their Relationships with Food through Myths, Metaphors and Storytelling* (Gurze Books, 1996).

21. Dr. Clarissa Pinkola Estés, *Women Who Run with the Wolves: Myths and Stories of the Wild Woman Archetype* (Ballantine, 1992), pp. 265–257.

22. Rebecca Orleane, *The Return of the Feminine: Honoring the Cycles of Nature*, p. 32. See also Edward Dewey and Edwin Dakin, *Cycles: The Science of Prediction* (2010 [1947]); George Haralambie, "The Global Crisis and Cyclical Theory," *Theoretical and Applied Economics* XVIIII, no. 11, issue 564 (2011): 79–88.

23. Annabel Crabb, *The Wife Drought* (Penguin, 2014).

24. Mary Helen Immordino-Yang, Joanna A. Christodoulou, and Vanessa Singh, "Rest Is Not Idleness: Implications of the Brain's Default Mode for Human Development and Education," *Perspectives on Psychological Science* 7, no. 4 (July 2012): 352–364.

25. Dr. Carl Jung, *Letters of CG Jung, Volume I, 1906–1950*, edited by Gerhard Adler (Routledge, 2015).

26. Kevin Farrow, *The Psychology of the Body* (2006).

27. *The Old Farmer's Almanac* recommends the planting in the first half of the Moon cycle of flowers and vegetables that bear crops aboveground, and the planting of flowering bulbs and vegetables that bear crops belowground in the second half of the moon cycle. See http://www.almanac.com/content/planting-moons-phase-gardening-calendar. See also David Whitehouse, *The Moon: A Biography* (Headline Book Publishing, 2001).

28. Etty Hillesum, *An Interrupted Life: The Diaries of Etty Hillesum, 1941–1943* (Washington Square Press, 1985).

29. Farrow, *Psychology of the Body.*

30. Donnell Lefort, *The Esoteric Codex: Primordial Teachers* (EC Publishers, 2015), p. 34.

31. This was recounted to an anthropologist by a traditional Yolgnu man early in the 20th century: W. L. Warner, *A Black Civilization* (Harper, 1937).

32. Buddha wrote of the mind and body being interlinked: "If you wish to see why the body is the way it is, look at how you've been thinking for the past ten years. If you wish to see how your body will be in ten years' time, look at how you're thinking now." Buddha, 550 BCE, cited in Kevin Farrow, *Energy Medicine* (Winter, 2009). An early psychological proponent of this was William James, *The Principles of Psychology* (Holt, 1890). It is now a concept increasingly accepted by the medical profession. See, e.g., Dr. Christiane Northrup, *Women's Bodies, Women's Wisdom* (Piatkus Books, 1995) pp. 25–26.

33. Benjamin Baird, Jonathan Smallwood, Michael D. Mrazek, Julia W. Y. Kam, Michael S. Franklin, and Jonathan W. Schooler, "Inspired by Distraction: Mind Wandering Facilitates Creative Incubation," *Psychological Science* 23, no. 10 (August 2012): 1117–1122; Ap Dijksterhuis, Maarten W. Bos, Loran F. Nordgren, and Rick B. van Baaren, "On Making the Right Choice: The Deliberation-without-Attention Effect," *Science*, New Series, 311, no. 5763 (February 17, 2006): 1005–1007; Mary Helen Immordino-Yang, Joanna A. Christodoulou, and Vanessa Singh, "Rest Is Not Idleness: Implications of the Brain's Default Mode for Human Development and Education," *Perspectives on Psychological Science* 7, no. 4 (2012): 352–364.

34. K. Anders Ericsson, Ralf T. Krampe, and Clemens Tesch-Römer, "The Role of Deliberate Practice in the Acquisition of Expert Performance," *Psychological Review* 100, no. 3, (July 1993): 363–406.

35. James Doty, *Into the Magic Shop* (Avery, 2015): 50.

36. R. Jerath, J. W. Edry, V. A. Barnes, and V. Jerath, "Physiology of Long Pranayamic Breathing: Neural Respiratory Elements May Provide a Mechanism That Explains How Slow Deep Breathing Shifts the Autonomic Nervous System," *Medical Hypotheses* 67, no. 3 (2006): 566–571. Ravinder Jerath, Molly W. Crawford, Vernon A. Barnes, and Kyler Harden, "Self-Regulation of Breathing as a Primary Treatment for Anxiety," *Applied Psychophysiology and Biofeedback* 40 (2015): 107–111; Volker Busch, Walter Magerl, Uwe Kern, Joachim Haas, Göran Hajak, and Peter Eichhammer, "The Effect of Deep and Slow Breathing on Pain Perception, Autonomic Activity, and Mood Processing: An Experimental Study," *American Academy of Pain Medicine* 13, no. 2 (2011): 215–228; Ravinder Jerath and Vernon A. Barnes, "Augmentation of Mind-Body Therapy and Role of Deep Slow Breathing," *Journal of Complementary and Integrative Medicine* 6, no. 1 (January 2009): 566–571.

37. William James, *The Principles of Psychology* (Holt, 1890).

38. George, *Mysteries of the Dark Moon*, pp. 15–16.

39. P. R. Clance and S. A. Imes, "The Impostor Phenomenon in High Achieving Women: Dynamics and Therapeutic Intervention," *Psychotherapy: Theory, Research, and Practice* 15, no. 3 (1978) 241–247.

40. Amy Cuddy, *Presence* (Little, Brown, 2015).

41. "Hillary Clinton, Melissa Harris-Perry and the Opposite of Imposter Syndrome," Huffington Post (March 27, 2016): www.huffingtonpost.com/anna-kegler/hillary-clinton-and-the-opposite-of-imposter-syndrome_b_9553190.html.

42. Marion Woodman and Elinor Dickson, *Dancing in the Flames: The Dark Goddess in the Transformation of Consciousness* (Shambhala, 1997), p. 58.

43. Mariana Caplan, *Eyes Wide Open: Cultivating Discernment on the Spiritual Path* (Sounds True, 2009).

44. Woodman and Dickson, *Dancing in the Flames*, p. 62.

45. Louisa May Alcott, *Good Wives* (Cosimo, 2010).

46. Viktor E. Frankl, *Man's Search for Meaning*, translated by Ilse Lasch with a foreword by Harold S. Kushner (Beacon Press, 1946).

47. Michael Philp, Sarah Egan, and Robert Kane, "Perfectionism, Over Commitment to Work, and Burnout in Employees Seeking Workplace Counseling," *Australian Journal of Psychology* (2012); Els van der Helm, MSc; Ninad Gujar, MSc; and Matthew P. Walker, PhD, "Sleep Deprivation Impairs the Accurate Recognition of Human Emotions." On the far end of the scale, perfectionism can result in heightened suicide risk: Gordon L. Flett, Paul L. Hewitt, and Marin J. Heisel, "The Destructiveness of Perfectionism Revisited: Implications for the Assessment of Suicide Risk and the Prevention of Suicide," *Review of General Psychology* 18, no. 3 (September 2014): 156–172.

48.	Dr. Brené Brown, *Rising Strong* (Random House, 2015).

49.	Virginia Woolf, *The Waves* (Macmillan Collectors Library, 2005 [1931]), p. 86.

50.	George, *Mysteries of the Dark Moon*, pp. 15–16.

51.	George, *Mysteries of the Dark Moon*, p. 12.

52.	Edain McCoy, *Magick & Rituals of the Moon* (Llewellyn Publications, 2001), p. 201.

53.	Philip M. Ullrich and Susan K. Lutgendorf, "Journaling about Stressful Events: Effects of Cognitive Processing and Emotional Expression," *Annals of Behavioural Medicine* 24, no. 3 (2002): 244–250.

54.	Richard Stephens, John Atkins, and Andrew Kingston, "Swearing as a Response to Pain" *NeuroReport* 20 (2009): 1056–1060.

55.	Benjamin P. Chapman, Kevin Fiscella, Ichiro Kawachi, Paul Duberstein, and Peter Muennig, "Emotion Suppression and Mortality Risk over a 12-Year Follow-up," *Journal of Psychosomatic Research* 75, no. 4 (October 2013): 381–385.

56.	Thomas Gilovich, Amit Kumar, and Lily Jampol, "A Wonderful Life: Experiential Consumption and the Pursuit of Happiness," *Journal of Consumer Psychology* 25, no. 1, (January 2015): 152–165.

57.	Julie Sheldon, *The Blessing of Tears* (Hymns Ancient & Modern Ltd, 2004), pp. 6–7. See also Ad Vingerhoets, *Why Only Humans Weep: Unravelling the Mysteries of Tears* (Oxford University Press, 2013).

58.	X. D. Martin and M. C. Brennan, "Serotonin in Human Tears," *European Journal of Ophthalmology* 4, no. 3 (July–September 1994): 159–165.

59.	Judith Orloff, *Emotional Freedom: Liberate Yourself from Negative Emotions and Transform Your Life* (Harmony Books, 2010), p. 293.

60. Maya Angelou, *Maya Angelou: Her Words* (Lulu Press, 2014).

61. George, *Mysteries of the Dark Moon*, pp. 15–16.

62. Estés, *Women Who Run with the Wolves*, p. 79.

63. Jonah Paquette, *Real Happiness: Proven Paths for Contentment, Peace and Well-Being* (Pesi Publishing and Media, 2015), p. 39. Paquette cites studies by McCullough et al. (2002) and Bartlett (2006).

64. Maureen Murdock, *The Heroine's Journey* (Shambhala, 1990).

65. See Woodman and Dickson *Dancing in the Flames*, p. 62. Woodman and Dickson write that "part of the feminine task in its journey toward wholeness is a recognition and reception of masculine spirit."

66. Dan P. McAdams and Jen Guo, "Narrating the Generative Life," *Psychological Science* 26, no. 4 (April 2015): 475–483. See also the discussion in Kat McGowan, "Silicon Phoenix," *Aeon* (May 2, 2016): https://aeon.co/essays/how-silicon-valley-rewrote-america-s-redemption-narrative.

67. Dr. Brené Brown, *The Gifts of Imperfection: Let Go of Who You Think You're Supposed to Be and Embrace Who You Are* (Hazelden Publications, 2010), p. 20.

68. The first study to demonstrate the so-called "McClintock effect" was Martha K. McClintock, "Menstrual Synchrony and Suppression," *Nature* (January 22, 1971): 229, 244–245. See also Martha K. McClintock, "On the Nature of Mammalian and Human Pheromones," *Annals of the New York Academy of Sciences* 855 (November 1998): 390–392.

69. George, *Mysteries of the Dark Moon*, pp. 15–16.

70. Chögyam Trungpa Rinpoche, *The Collected Works of Chögyam Trungpa: Volume 8: Great Eastern Sun Shambhala Selected Writings* (Shambhala Press), p. 115.

71. George, *Mysteries of the Dark Moon*, pp. 15–19.

72. George, *Mysteries of the Dark Moon*, p. 6.

73. Virginia Woolf, *A Writer's Diary* (Houghton Mifflin Harcourt, 2003).

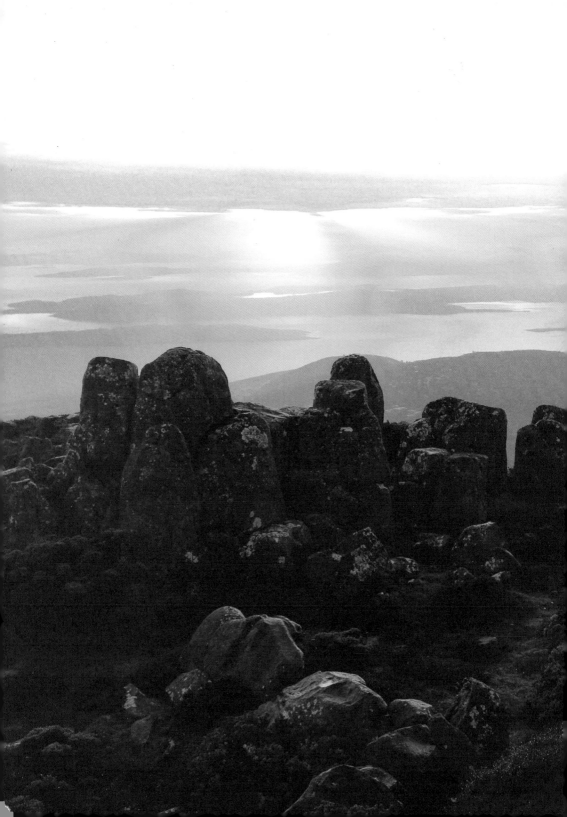